Complementary and Alternative Medicine

IN THE UNITED STATES

Committee on the Use of Complementary and Alternative Medicine
by the American Public
Board on Health Promotion and Disease Prevention

INSTITUTE OF MEDICINE
OF THE NATIONAL ACADEMIES

THE NATIONAL ACADEMIES PRESS
Washington, D.C.
www.nap.edu

THE NATIONAL ACADEMIES PRESS 500 Fifth Street, N.W. Washington, DC 20001

NOTICE: The project that is the subject of this report was approved by the Governing Board of the National Research Council, whose members are drawn from the councils of the National Academy of Sciences, the National Academy of Engineering, and the Institute of Medicine. The members of the committee responsible for the report were chosen for their special competences and with regard for appropriate balance.

This study was supported by Contract No. 200N01-OD-4-2139 between the National Academy of Sciences and the Agency for Health Care Research and Quality, National Institutes of Health. Any opinions, findings, conclusions, or recommendations expressed in this publication are those of the author(s) and do not necessarily reflect the view of the organizations or agencies that provided support for this project.

Library of Congress Cataloging-in-Publication Data

Institute of Medicine (U.S.). Committee on the Use of Complementary and Alternative Medicine by the American Public.

Complementary and alternative medicine in the United States / Committee on the Use of Complementary and Alternative Medicine by the American Public, Board on Health Promotion and Disease Prevention.

    p. ; cm.

Includes bibliographical references and index.

ISBN 0-309-09270-1 (hardcover)

1. Alternative medicine—United States.

[DNLM: 1. Complementary Therapies—United States. 2. Biomedical Research—United States. 3. Health Policy—United States. WB 890 I59 2004] I. Title.

R733.I5633 2004

615.5′0973—dc22

                   2004029011

Additional copies of this report are available from the National Academies Press, 500 Fifth Street, N.W., Lockbox 285, Washington, DC 20055; (800) 624-6242 or (202) 334-3313 (in the Washington metropolitan area); Internet, http://www.nap.edu.

For more information about the Institute of Medicine, visit the IOM home page at: **www.iom.edu.**

Cover design by Tim and Karin Martin.

The serpent has been a symbol of long life, healing, and knowledge among almost all cultures and religions since the beginning of recorded history. The serpent adopted as a logotype by the Institute of Medicine is a relief carving from ancient Greece, now held by the Staatliche Museen in Berlin.

"Knowing is not enough; we must apply.
Willing is not enough; we must do."
—Goethe

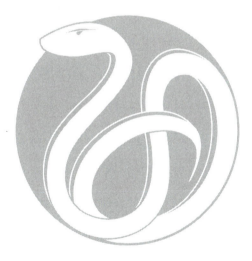

INSTITUTE OF MEDICINE
OF THE NATIONAL ACADEMIES

Adviser to the Nation to Improve Health

THE NATIONAL ACADEMIES
Advisers to the Nation on Science, Engineering, and Medicine

The **National Academy of Sciences** is a private, nonprofit, self-perpetuating society of distinguished scholars engaged in scientific and engineering research, dedicated to the furtherance of science and technology and to their use for the general welfare. Upon the authority of the charter granted to it by the Congress in 1863, the Academy has a mandate that requires it to advise the federal government on scientific and technical matters. Dr. Bruce M. Alberts is president of the National Academy of Sciences.

The **National Academy of Engineering** was established in 1964, under the charter of the National Academy of Sciences, as a parallel organization of outstanding engineers. It is autonomous in its administration and in the selection of its members, sharing with the National Academy of Sciences the responsibility for advising the federal government. The National Academy of Engineering also sponsors engineering programs aimed at meeting national needs, encourages education and research, and recognizes the superior achievements of engineers. Dr. Wm. A. Wulf is president of the National Academy of Engineering.

The **Institute of Medicine** was established in 1970 by the National Academy of Sciences to secure the services of eminent members of appropriate professions in the examination of policy matters pertaining to the health of the public. The Institute acts under the responsibility given to the National Academy of Sciences by its congressional charter to be an adviser to the federal government and, upon its own initiative, to identify issues of medical care, research, and education. Dr. Harvey V. Fineberg is president of the Institute of Medicine.

The **National Research Council** was organized by the National Academy of Sciences in 1916 to associate the broad community of science and technology with the Academy's purposes of furthering knowledge and advising the federal government. Functioning in accordance with general policies determined by the Academy, the Council has become the principal operating agency of both the National Academy of Sciences and the National Academy of Engineering in providing services to the government, the public, and the scientific and engineering communities. The Council is administered jointly by both Academies and the Institute of Medicine. Dr. Bruce M. Alberts and Dr. Wm. A. Wulf are chair and vice chair, respectively, of the National Research Council.

www.national-academies.org

Mark Nichter, PhD, MPH, Professor of Anthropology, Professor of Family and Community Medicine, Professor of Public Health, University of Arizona

Bernard Rosof, MD, FACP, Senior Vice President for Corporate Relations and Health Affairs, North Shore Long Island Jewish Health System

Harold Sox, MD, FACP, Editor, *Annals of Internal Medicine*

Liaison to Board on Health Promotion and Disease Prevention

Ellen Gritz, PhD, Professor and Chair, Frank T. McGraw Memorial Chair in the Study of Cancer, and Department of Behavioral Science, The University of Texas M.D. Anderson Cancer Center

Committee Consultant

Michael H. Cohen, JD, MBA, MFA, Assistant Professor of Medicine, Harvard Medical School, and Attorney-at-Law

Staff

Lyla M. Hernandez, MPH, Study Director

Kysa Christie, Senior Program Associate

Makisha Wiley, Senior Program Assistant

Rose Marie Martinez, ScD, Director, Board on Health Promotion and Disease Prevention

Preface

Complementary and alternative medicine (CAM) therapies, by whatever name they are called, have existed from antiquity. Recognition of the widespread use of CAM by the people of the United States has given new emphasis to the need to better understand the effects of these treatments from the perspective of personal and public health. To provide a rational, effective, efficient, and personally satisfactory health care system, it is important and useful to know who is using CAM therapies and why, how the public obtains information about CAM and how credible that information is, why many users of CAM do not inform their physicians about such use, just what CAM is, and whether these therapies are safe and effective.

It is only relatively recently, however, that there has been a serious general interest in the United States in investigating and evaluating these therapies. In 1992 the U.S. Congress established the Office of Alternative Medicine (OAM) within the National Institutes of Health (NIH) to begin to develop a baseline of information on CAM use in the United States. In 1999 the Congress elevated OAM to the National Center for Complementary and Alternative Medicine and appropriated $48.9 million to carry out work directly related to CAM. Other institutes of NIH and other federal agencies also engaged in the effort and by 2003, 19 institutes and centers within NIH were collectively spending $315.5 million on CAM-related research and other activities.

This report was commissioned in September 2002, when 16 NIH institutes, centers, and offices plus the Agency for Healthcare Research and Quality asked the Institute of Medicine to convene a study committee to explore scientific, policy, and practice questions that arise from the significant and increasing use of CAM therapies by the American public. Specifically, this study was asked to

1. Describe the use of CAM therapies by the American public and provide a comprehensive overview, to the extent that data are available, of the therapies in widespread use, the populations that use them, and what is known about how they are provided.
2. Identify the major scientific, policy, and practice issues related to CAM research and to the translation of validated therapies into conventional medical practice.
3. Develop conceptual models or frameworks to guide public- and private-sector decision making as research and practice communities confront the challenges of conducting research on CAM, translating research findings into practice, and addressing the distinct policy and practice barriers inherent in that translation.

Furthermore, the committee was asked to explore several issues, including

• the methodological difficulties in the conduct of rigorous research on CAM therapies and how these relate to issues in regulation and practice, with exploration of the options that can be used to address the difficulties identified.
• the shortage of highly skilled practitioners who are able to participate in scientific inquiry that meets NIH guidelines and who have access to the institutions where such research is conducted.
• the shortage of receptive, integrated research environments and the barriers to developing multidisciplinary teams that include CAM and conventional medical practitioners.
• the availability of standardized and well-characterized materials and practices to be studied and incorporated, when appropriate, into practice.
• the existing decision-making models used to determine whether or not to incorporate new therapies and practices into conventional medicine, including evidence thresholds.
• the applicability of these decision-making models to CAM therapies and practices; that is, do they form good precedents for decisions relating to regulation, accreditation, or integration of CAM therapies?
• identification and analysis of successful approaches to the incorporation of CAM into health professions education.
• the impact of current regulations and legislation on CAM research and integration.

Committee membership was chosen to represent the most salient perspectives and competences, since there was no possibility that all or even most of the interest groups could be represented. Members included providers of CAM and conventional health care as well as analysts, observers, and managers of CAM and conventional health care systems. To ensure effective input from CAM providers, the committee established a working liaison group composed of 35 leaders of CAM and conventional medical disciplines and held a number of formal and informal interchanges with these groups.

The committee proceeded to educate and inform itself through a systematic review of the extensive relevant literature, a series of expert presentations, discussions, and public comments in open meetings, and focused interchange and deliberation in committee meetings. The work of the committee was especially informed by discussions and a paper on experimental design written for the committee by Naihua Duan, Joel Braslow, Alison Hamilton Brown, Ted J. Kaptchuk, and Louise E. Tallen. The agendas and participants in the public meetings are listed in Appendix G.

As described more extensively in Chapter 1 of the report, the committee deliberated at length concerning whether and how to define CAM most usefully for the purpose of this report. All proposed definitions were imprecise, ambiguous, or otherwise subject to misinterpretation. Judging that a definition was necessary, for the purposes of this report the committee adopted the definition stated on page 19. Several important caveats need to be understood to interpret correctly the committee's meaning of statements concerning CAM in this report. The definition is necessarily imprecise and nonlimiting since it is based in part on the implied intended purpose of the practitioner and the user (i.e., improvement of health outcomes) and in part on exclusion from a category (the dominant health care system) that itself is not precisely defined and that changes substantially over time.

The term *CAM*, as used in this report, encompasses a large, diverse, and changing set of "systems, modalities, and practices and their theories and beliefs." The diversity of practice within CAM is so great that there are few, if any, generalizations that apply equally to all systems, modalities, and practices defined as CAM. When the term CAM is used in this report, it is not intended to include all CAM practices equally but, rather, to refer to a substantial group of CAM practices.

The work of the committee began with the question, what do patients and health professionals need to know to make good decisions about the use of health care interventions, including CAM? Of primary importance in making decisions about whether to use specific CAM therapies is determining that they are safe and effective. There are extremes of belief about effectiveness; for some individuals, no other evidence than hearsay or their own experience or knowledge is necessary to determine that a CAM therapy is effective. For others, no evidence of any quality or quantity is sufficient to prove CAM effective. This report will please neither of those extremes.

Recognizing that all scientific conclusions are tentative, the committee adopted proven and conventional standards of scientific evidence as the basis for judgments of the safety and effectiveness of both CAM and conventional medicine.

The widespread use of CAM has focused attention on the need to find answers to the numerous questions surrounding such use, questions such as who is using CAM therapies and why, how does the public obtain information about CAM and how credible is that information, why aren't users of CAM informing their physicians about such use, just what is CAM and are these therapies safe and effective?

A significant portion of this report is devoted to an examination and analysis of evidence: what it is, how we obtain it, and how it is used by various stakeholders to make decisions. Methodological challenges are examined, and innovative study designs are discussed. Existing evidence about the effectiveness of some CAM therapies is reviewed and gaps in our knowledge are identified. Input from the liaison panel was particularly important as the committee explored the issue of evidence and how we know what we know.

The report also addresses a number of issues related to the integration of CAM and conventional medicine, including how a therapy moves from a new idea to an accepted practice, a framework for advising patients about CAM, and approaches to integration. The committee concluded that the goal should be the provision of comprehensive medical care that is based on the best scientific evidence available regarding benefits and harm, that encourages patients to share in decision making about therapeutic options, and that promotes choices in care that can include CAM therapies, when appropriate. Our challenge was to eliminate parochial bias and to apply the best-available means of assessment of safety and effectiveness adapted to particular clinical circumstances of both CAM and conventional medicine. In this way we will be able to ensure that we are making informed, reasoned, and knowledge-based decisions about the safety, effectiveness, and use of CAM in health care.

On behalf of every member of the committee, I want to express our unbounded respect and appreciation for the wisdom, industry, and judgment that Lyla Hernandez put into this study. At many critical junctures she kept the committee on track; and she was regularly a source of important ideas, data, and experts. The study would not have been completed without her gracious perseverance. We also want to thank Kysa Christie, who provided thoughtful and invaluable research support. Ms. Christie identified, evaluated, and synthesized background information and issues throughout the committee's deliberations. And we thank Makisha Wiley, who expertly managed our administrative, meeting, and travel needs.

Stuart Bondurant, *Committee Chair*

Acknowledgments

Throughout the past two years, the IOM Committee on the Use of Complementary and Alternative Medicine (CAM) by the American Public was fortunate to interact with many individuals interested in the role of CAM in the United States and willing to share their expertise, time and thoughts with the committee.

The study sponsors at the NIH Institutes and Centers and the Agency for Healthcare Research and Quality willingly responded to questions and provided information on historical and ongoing projects related to complementary and alternative medicine. In particular, the committee wishes to thank Stephen E. Straus, Linda W. Engel, and Wendy Smith.

Speakers at the five public meetings provided a broad overview of the field of CAM and its interaction with conventional medicine, as well as providing specific information about CAM. We would like to thank those speakers: Joseph Betz, Timothy Birdsall, Opher Caspi, Garrett Cuneo, Steven Dentali, George DeVries, Claude Gagnon, Harley Goldberg, James Gordon, Milton Hammerly, Aviad Haramati, William R. Hazzard, Dilip Jeste, Wayne Jonas, Mary Jo Kreitzer, Lee Lipsenthal, John Melnychuk, Will Morris, David Morrison, Donald Novey, Willo Pequegnat, Rowena Richter, Lawrence Smith, and Stephen E. Straus.

In addition to the invited presentations, the committee wishes to acknowledge the contributions of those individuals who provided their insights during public comment sessions: Susan Bonfield Herschkowitz, Ardith Dentzer, Victoria Goldsten, William Lauretti, John Longhurst, Antonio C. Martinez II, Randall Neustaedter, Anthony Rosner, Harry Swope, Marissa Valeri, Kelly Welch, and James Winterstein.

Understanding and exploring research methods were crucial to the committee's deliberations and the committee is indebted to Naihua Duan and his collaborators, Joel Braslow, Alison Hamilton Brown, Ted J. Kaptchuk, and Louise E. Tallen who were commissioned to write a paper on the strengths and limitations of clinical research. Thanks also go to the reviewers of that paper Elizabeth Barrett-Connor, Wayne Jonas, Roger Lewis, and Lee Sechrest. The committee would also like to thank Eric Manheimer for his contributions about emerging evidence in Chapter 5.

Finally, a unique and informative component of the committee's information gathering processes was the liaison panel with representatives from professional organizations in both conventional, and complementary and alternative medicine. Members of the liaison panel who met with, and provided input to the committee included: John Balletto, Timothy Birdsall, John P. Borneman, Gene C. Bruno, Clair Callan, Edward H. Chapman, Council on Homeopathic Education, Bryn Clark, Robert M. Duggan, Charlotte Eliopoulis, Joyce Frye, Milt Hammerly, Mark Houston, Herb Jacobs, Reiner Kremer, William Lauretti, John Lunstroth, Robert S. McCaleb, Alice McCormick, Matthew McCoy, Walter J. McDonald, William McCarthy, Ana C. Micka, David Molony, Will Morris, Wayne Mylin, Hiroshi Nakazawa, Randall Neustaedter, Martha S. O'Connor, Carole Ostendorf, Lawrence B. Palevsky, John Pan, Reed Phillips, Marcia Prenguber, Iris Ratowsky, Cynthia K. Reeser, David Rosengard, Cynthia Reeser, Rustum Roy, William D. Rutenberg, David M. Sale, Arnold Sandlow, Edward Shalts, Thomas Shepherd, Harry Swope, John Tooker, Richard Walls, Don Warren, Kathryn A. Weiner, Julian Whitaker, James F. Winterstein, Jackie Wootton.

Reviewers

This report has been reviewed in draft form by individuals chosen for their diverse perspectives and technical expertise, in accordance with procedures approved by the NRC's Report Review Committee. The purpose of this independent review is to provide candid and critical comments that will assist the institution in making its published report as sound as possible and to ensure that the report meets institutional standards for objectivity, evidence, and responsiveness to the study charge. The review comments and draft manuscript remain confidential to protect the integrity of the deliberative process. We wish to thank the following individuals for their review of this report:

Donald Berry, The University of Texas M.D. Anderson Cancer Center
Timothy C. Birdsall, Cancer Treatment Centers of America
Robert Boruch, Graduate School of Education, University of Pennsylvania
Howard Brody, Center for Ethics and Humanities in the Life Sciences, Michigan State University
Phil B. Fontanarosa, *The Journal of the American Medical Association*
Janet Kahn, Department of Psychiatry, University of Vermont
Mary Anne Koda-Kimble, School of Pharmacy, University of California, San Francisco
Christine Laine, *Annals of Internal Medicine,* and American College of Physicians
Roger J. Lewis, Department of Emergency Medicine, Harbor-University of California at Los Angeles Medical Center

William Meeker, Palmer Center for Chiropractic Research, Palmer
  Chiropractic University Foundation
Anne Nedrow, Women's Primary Care and Integrative Medicine, Oregon
  Health & Science University
Susan Scrimshaw, School of Public Health, University of Illinois at
  Chicago
Michael Trujillo, Department of Family and Community Medicine,
  University of New Mexico Health Sciences Center

Although the reviewers listed above have provided many constructive comments and suggestions, they were not asked to endorse the conclusions or recommendations nor did they see the final draft of the report before its release. The review of this report was overseen by Dan G. Blazer, J.P. Gibbons Professor of Psychiatry, Duke University Medical Center, and Henry W. Riecken, Professor of Behavioral Sciences, Emeritus, University of Pennsylvania. Appointed by the National Research Council and the Institute of Medicine, they were responsible for making certain that an independent examination of this report was carried out in accordance with institutional procedures and that all review comments were carefully considered. Responsibility for the final content of this report rests entirely with the authoring committee and the institution.

Contents

Complementary and Alternative Medicine

IN THE UNITED STATES

Executive Summary

Americans' use of complementary and alternative medicine (CAM)—approaches such as chiropractic or acupuncture—is widespread. More than a third of American adults report using some form of CAM, with total visits to CAM providers each year now exceeding those to primary-care physicians. An estimated 15 million adults take herbal remedies or high-dose vitamins along with prescription drugs. It all adds up to annual out-of-pocket costs for CAM that are estimated to exceed $27 billion.

Friends confer with friends about CAM remedies for specific problems, CAM-related stories appear frequently in the print and broadcast media, and the Internet is replete with CAM information. Many hospitals, managed care plans, and conventional practitioners are incorporating CAM therapies into their practices, and schools of medicine, nursing, and pharmacy are beginning to teach about CAM.

CAM's influence is substantial yet much remains unknown about these therapies, particularly with regard to scientific studies that might convincingly demonstrate the value of individual therapies. Against this background the National Center for Complementary and Alternative Medicine (NCCAM), 15 other centers and institutes of the National Institutes of Health (NIH), and the Agency for Healthcare Research and Quality commissioned the Institute of Medicine (IOM) to convene a committee that would

- Describe the use of CAM therapies by the American public and provide a comprehensive overview, to the extent that data are available, of the therapies in widespread use, the populations that use them, and what is known about how they are provided.

- Identify major scientific, policy, and practice issues related to CAM research and to the translation of validated therapies into conventional medical practice.

- Develop conceptual models or frameworks to guide public- and private-sector decisionmaking as research and practice communities increasingly conduct research on CAM, translate the research findings into practice, and address the barriers that may impede such translation.

TOWARD COMMON RESEARCH GROUND

Decisions about the use of specific CAM therapies should primarily depend on whether they have been shown to be safe and effective. But this is easier said than done, as there are extremes of belief about what counts as evidence. For some individuals, evidence limited to their own experience or knowledge is all that is necessary as proof that a CAM therapy is successful; for others, *no* amount of evidence is sufficient. This report will please neither of those extremes.

There are unproven ideas of all kinds, stemming from CAM and conventional medicine alike, and the committee believes that the same principles and standards of evidence should apply regardless of a treatment's origin. Study results may then move useful therapies from unproven ideas into evidence-based practice.

The goal should be the provision of comprehensive care that respects contributions from all sources. Such care requires decisions based on the results of scientific inquiry, which in turn can lead to new information that results in improvements in patient care.

This report's core message is therefore as follows: **The committee recommends that the same principles and standards of evidence of treatment effectiveness apply to all treatments, whether currently labeled as conventional medicine or CAM. Implementing this recommendation requires that investigators use and develop as necessary common methods, measures, and standards for the generation and interpretation of evidence necessary for making decisions about the use of CAM and conventional therapies.**

The committee acknowledges that the characteristics of some CAM therapies—such as variable practitioner approaches, customized treatments, "bundles" (combinations) of treatments, and hard-to-measure outcomes— are difficult to incorporate into treatment-effectiveness studies. These characteristics are not unique to CAM, but they are more frequently found in CAM than in conventional therapies. The effects of mass-produced, essentially identical prescription drugs, for example, are somewhat easier to study than those of Chinese herbal medicines tailored to the needs of individual patients.

But while randomized controlled trials (RCTs) remain the "gold standard" of evidence for treatment efficacy, other study designs can be used to provide information about effectiveness when RCTs cannot be done or when their results may not be generalizable to the real world of CAM practice. These innovative designs include:

- *Preference RCTs*: trials that include randomized and non-randomized arms, which then permit comparisons between patients who chose a particular treatment and those who were randomly assigned to it
- *Observational and cohort studies*, which involve the identification of patients who are eligible for study and who may receive a specified treatment, but are not randomly assigned to the specified treatment as part of the study
- *Case-control studies*, which involve identifying patients who have good or bad outcomes, then "working back" to find aspects of treatment associated with those different outcomes
- *Studies of bundles of therapies*: analyses of the effectiveness, as a whole, of particular packages of treatments
- *Studies that specifically incorporate, measure, or account for placebo or expectation effects*: patients' hopes, emotional states, energies, and other self-healing processes are not considered extraneous but are included as part of the therapy's main "mechanisms of action"
- *Attribute-treatment interaction analyses*: a way of accounting for differences in effectiveness outcomes among patients within a study and among different studies of varying design

Given limited available funding, prioritization is necessary regarding which CAM therapies to evaluate. The following criteria could be used to help make this determination:

- A biologically plausible mechanism exists for the intervention, but the science base on which plausibility is judged is a work in progress.
- Research could plausibly lead to the discovery of biological mechanisms of disease or treatment effect.
- The condition is highly prevalent (e.g., diabetes mellitus).
- The condition causes a heavy burden of suffering.
- The potential benefit is great.
- Some evidence that the intervention is effective already exists.
- Some evidence exists that there are safety concerns.

- The research design is feasible, and research will likely yield an unambiguous result.
- The target condition or the intervention is important enough to have been detected by existing population-surveillance mechanisms.

A therapy should not be excluded from consideration because it does not meet any one particular criterion—say, biological plausibility. However, the absence of such a mechanism will inevitably raise the level of skepticism about the potential effectiveness of the treatment (whether conventional or CAM). Moreover, the amount of basic research needed to justify funding for clinical studies of the treatment, and the level of evidence from those studies that is needed to consider the treatment as "established," will both increase under such circumstances.

A NEW POSITION ON DIETARY SUPPLEMENTS

The committee has taken a similarly pragmatic approach to dietary supplements, which have become a prominent part of American popular health culture but continue to present unique regulatory, safety, and efficacy challenges.

Under the Dietary Supplement Health and Education Act of 1994—the capstone, thus far, of herbal-medicine regulation—the Food and Drug Administration (FDA) was authorized to establish good-manufacturing-practice regulations specific to dietary supplements. But the Act did not subject supplements to the same safety precautions that apply to prescription and over-the-counter medications. Instead, it designated that supplements be regulated like foods, a crucial distinction that exempted manufacturers from conducting premarket safety and efficacy testing. Similarly, FDA's regulatory-approval process—which would be standard operating procedure if supplements had been classified as drugs—was eliminated, thereby limiting the agency to a reactive, postmarketing role.

The committee is concerned about the quality of dietary supplements in the United States. Product reliability is low, and because patent protection is not available for natural substances there is little incentive for manufacturers to invest resources in improving product standardization. Yet reliable and standardized supplements are needed not only for consumer protection but also for research on safety and efficacy. Without consistent products, research is extremely difficult to conduct or generalize. And without high-quality research, medical practitioners cannot make evidence-based recommendations to help guide patients.

Therefore **the committee recommends that the U.S. Congress and federal agencies, in consultation with industry, research scientists, consumers, and other stakeholders, amend the Dietary Supplement Health and Educa-**

tion Act of 1994 and the current regulatory scheme for dietary supplements, with emphasis on strengthening:

- Seed-to-shelf quality-control (based on standards for each step of the manufacturing process—from planting to growth, harvest, extraction, and screening for impurities),
  - Accuracy and comprehensiveness in labeling and other disclosures,
  - Enforcement efforts against inaccurate and misleading claims,
  - Research into how consumers use supplements,
- Incentives for privately funded research into the efficacies of products and brands, and
  - Consumer protection against all potential hazards.

FILLING THE GAPS

Evidence of the safety and efficacy of individual CAM treatments is essential, but it represents just one facet of the research that is needed. For example, there is a paucity of clinical research that compares CAM therapies with each other or with conventional interventions. Very little research has been done on the cost-effectiveness of CAM. And although there is great opportunity for scientific discovery in the study of CAM treatments, it is an opportunity largely missed.

Such investigations are hindered by shortages of established scientists engaged in CAM research, which tends to involve subject matter beyond the conventional scientist's knowledge base. CAM also needs a cadre of new junior researchers. While major U.S. health-sciences campuses have long offered training in basic and clinical research for conventional medicine, the challenge is to induce these schools to embrace CAM research as well. One approach might be to add specific CAM content to conventional-medicine postdoctoral training programs.

Furthermore, CAM research will benefit from the contributions of more than one discipline. In addition to providers who have specialized knowledge of CAM treatments and methodologists who can address the challenges inherent in CAM study design, investigators with backgrounds in fields such as psychology, sociology, anthropology, economics, genetics, pharmacology, neuroscience, health services, and health policy can make important contributions. Interdisciplinary teams, grouped into "critical masses" at various locations, will be favorably positioned to probe the many factors that influence individuals to use CAM treatments and that determine the outcomes of those treatments.

Research on CAM is inextricably linked to practice. CAM therapies are already in widespread use today; it is reasonable to attempt to evaluate the outcomes of that use, and in the practice setting one can focus on research that answers questions about how therapies function in the "real world" where patients vary, often have a number of health problems, and are using multiple therapies. Practice-based research addresses real world practice issues and facilitates adoption of practice changes that are based on research results.

To address these gaps, **the committee recommends that the National Institutes of Health (NIH) and other public agencies provide the support necessary to:**

• **develop and implement a sentinel surveillance system** (composed of selected sites able to collect and report data on patterns of use of CAM and conventional medicine); **practice-based research networks** (defined by the Agency for Healthcare Research and Quality as "a group of ambulatory practices devoted principally to the primary care of patients, affiliated with each other [and often with an academic or professional organization] in order to investigate questions related to community-based practice"); **and CAM research centers to facilitate the work of the networks** (by collecting and analyzing information from national surveys, identifying important questions, designing studies, coordinating data collection and analysis, and providing training in research and other areas).

• **include questions relevant to CAM on federally funded health care surveys** (e.g., the National Health Interview Survey) and in ongoing longitudinal cohort studies (e.g., the Nurses' Health Study and Framingham Heart Study).

• **implement periodic comprehensive, representative national surveys** to assess the changes in prevalence, patterns, perceptions, and costs of therapy use (both CAM and conventional), with oversampling of ethnic minorities.

INTEGRATING CAM AND CONVENTIONAL MEDICINE

Even as CAM and conventional medicine each maintain their identities, traditions, and practitioners, integration of CAM and conventional medicine is occuring in many settings. Hospitals are offering CAM therapies, a growing number of physicians are using them in their private practices, integrative-medicine centers (many with close ties to medical schools and teaching hospitals) are being established, and health maintenance organizations and insurance companies are covering CAM.

Cancer treatment centers in particular often use CAM therapies in combination with conventional approaches. For example, the Memorial Sloan-Kettering Cancer Center has developed an Integrative Medicine Service that offers music therapy, massage, reflexology, and mind-body therapies. As the Website of the Dana Farber Cancer Institute's own Zakim Center for Integrated Therapies explains, "When patients integrate these therapies into their medical and surgical care, they are creating a more comprehensive treatment plan and helping their own bodies to regain health and vitality."

In response to the growing recognition of CAM therapies by conventional-medicine practitioners for their patients' care, the Federation of State Medical Boards of the United States has developed *Model Guidelines for the Use of Complementary and Alternative Therapies in Medical Practice.*

Other tools are also needed to aid conventional practitioners' decisionmaking about offering or recommending CAM, where patients might be referred, and what organizational structures are most appropriate for the delivery of integrated care. The committee believes that the overarching rubric for guiding the development of these tools should be the goal of providing comprehensive care that is safe, effective, interdisciplinary, and collaborative; is based on the best scientific evidence available; recognizes the importance of compassion and caring; and encourages patients to share in the choices of therapeutic options.

Studies show that patients frequently do not limit themselves to a single modality of care—they do not see CAM and conventional medicine as being mutually exclusive—and this pattern will probably continue and may even expand as evidence of therapies' effectiveness accumulates. Therefore it is important to understand how CAM and conventional medical treatments (and providers) interact with each other and to study models of how the two kinds of treatments can be provided in coordinated ways.

In that spirit, there is an urgent need for health systems research that focuses on identifying the elements of these integrative-medicine models, their outcomes, and whether they are cost-effective when compared to conventional practice.

The committee recommends that NIH and other public and private agencies sponsor research to compare:

- **the outcomes and costs of combinations of CAM and conventional medical treatments and models that deliver such care**
- **models of care delivery involving CAM practitioners alone, both CAM and conventional medical practitioners, and conventional practitioners alone. Outcome measures should include reproducibility, safety, cost-effectiveness, and research capacity**

Additionally, **the committee recommends that the Secretary of the U.S. Department of Health and Human Services and the Secretary of the U.S. Department of Veterans Affairs support research on integrated medical** care delivery, as well as the development of a research infrastructure within such organizations and clinical training programs to expand the number of providers able to work in integrated care.

The pursuit of such goals requires examination of the ethics of medicine, both in the provision of personal health services and the profession's advocacy for public health. Medicine is continuously shaped by larger social, cultural, and political forces, and the integration of CAM therapies is another juncture in this evolutionary process.

The ethical principles that guide conventional biomedical research should also be applied to CAM research. Legal and ethical issues often arise and sometimes conflict with use of CAM therapies because the decision facing a conventional practitioner or institution may engender a conflict between medical paternalism (the desire to protect patients from foolish or ill-informed, though voluntary decisions) and patient autonomy. The Model Guidelines noted above seek to establish greater balance between physician and patient preferences. In addition, a number of legal rules—including state licensure laws, precedents regarding malpractice liability and professional discipline, state and federal food and drug laws, and statutes on health care fraud—protect patients by enhancing quality assurance, offering enhanced access to therapies, and honoring medical pluralism in creating models of integrative care.

Without rejecting what has been of great value and service in the past, it is important that these ethical and legal norms be brought under critical scrutiny and evolve along with medicine's expanding knowledge base and the larger aims and meanings of medical practice. The integration of CAM therapies with conventional medicine requires that practitioners and researchers be open to diverse interpretations of health and healing, to finding innovative ways of obtaining evidence, and to expanding the medical knowledge base.

EDUCATING FOR IMPROVED CARE

Essential to conventional and CAM practitioners alike is education about the others' field. Conventional professionals in particular need enough CAM-related training, the committee believes, so that they can counsel patients in a manner consistent with high-quality comprehensive care. Therefore **the committee recommends that health profession schools (e.g., schools of medicine, nursing, pharmacy, and allied health) incorporate sufficient information about CAM into the standard curriculum at the undergraduate, graduate, and postgraduate levels to enable licensed professionals to competently advise their patients about CAM.**

Because the content and organization of an education initiative on CAM will vary from institution to institution, depending on the objectives of each program, there is no consensus on what should be taught and how to fit it into an already crowded set of courses. At Brown University School of Medicine, for example, the program includes didactic sessions in acupuncture, chiropractic, and massage therapy and an elective clinical experience; and variations exist at many of the other leading schools. Some of these initiatives have been aided by NCCAM's education projects, which aim to develop new ways of incorporating CAM into health-professional curricula and training programs.

CAM practitioners, for their part, need training that will enable them to participate as full partners and leaders in research so that studies may accurately reflect how CAM therapies are practiced. But many CAM institutions do not have an infrastructure for research or the financial resources to develop them. Training in research has not traditionally been part of CAM curricula, nor for the most part have practitioners' careers been dependent on publishing research findings. CAM institutions focus primarily on training for practice.

Strategic partnerships between CAM institutions, NIH, and health-sciences universities would help foster development of the necessary infrastructure; and NCCAM has already begun funding such partnerships. In addition, lessons can be learned from other fields, such as geriatrics and HIV/AIDS research, which have gone through processes relevant to CAM's current need to develop qualified researchers. In geriatrics, for instance, the establishment of centers of excellence at major academic health centers, foundation support for the development of curricula and partnerships, and continuing-education mechanisms such as summer institutes illustrate the importance of using multiple strategies to create an environment in which new science has been able to flourish.

The committee recommends that federal and state agencies, and private and corporate foundations, alone and in partnership, create models in research training for CAM practitioners.

Furthermore, both CAM research and the quality of CAM treatment would be fostered by the development of practice guidelines—what a 1992 IOM report defined as "systematically developed statements to assist practitioner and patient decisions about appropriate health care for specific clinical circumstances." Key to guideline development is the participation of those who will be most directly affected. This means that CAM practitioners, possibly through their own professional organizations, should formulate guidelines for their own therapies.

The committee recommends that national professional organizations for all CAM disciplines ensure the presence of training standards and develop practice guidelines. Health care professional licensing boards and

accrediting and certifying agencies (for both CAM and conventional medicine) should set competency standards in the appropriate use of both conventional medicine and CAM therapies, consistent with practitioners' scope of practice and standards of referral across health professions.

KNOWNS AND UNKNOWNS ABOUT CAM USE

Prevalence estimates for CAM use range from 30 percent to 62 percent of U.S. adults, depending on the definition of CAM. Women are more likely than men to seek CAM therapies, use appears to increase as education level increases, and there are varying patterns of use by race. Adults who undergo CAM therapies usually draw on more than one type, and they tend to do so in combination with conventional medical care—though a majority do not disclose the CAM use to their physicians, thereby incurring the risk, for example, of potential interactions between prescription drugs and CAM-related herbs. Studies of specific illnesses have documented the popularity of CAM for health problems that lack definitive cures, have unpredictable courses and prognoses, and are associated with substantial pain, discomfort, or medicinal side effects.

Existing surveys tell us little, however, about how CAM treatment is initiated (Does the patient unilaterally decide to use a therapy? Does a CAM or a conventional provider recommend the therapy?), and we have scant data about how the American public makes decisions about accessing CAM options. While there is an extensive literature on adherence to conventional treatment, there are virtually no data available on adherence to CAM treatment. This is an important issue given that any therapy, even if efficacious, may place users at risk of harm, or cause them to experience little or no effect, when used in the wrong way. Similarly, we have virtually no information about the extent to which the use of a CAM therapy may interfere with compliance in the use of conventional therapies, how people's self-administration of CAM therapies changes over time, and the factors that influence such change.

Moreover, there is little research on the public's perceptions of information as alternatively credible, marginal, or spurious; how people understand such information in terms of risks and benefits; and what they expect their providers to tell them. Because the few small studies that have occurred suggest that considerable misinformation is dispensed by vendors and on the Web, a closer monitoring of Websites, enhanced enforcement of the Dietary Supplement Health and Education Act as well as of Federal Trade Commission regulations, and the creation of a user-friendly authoritative Website on CAM modalities are needed.

As a means of remedying the dearth of information noted above, **the committee recommends that the National Institutes of Health and other** public or private agencies sponsor quantitative and qualitative research to examine:

- The social and cultural dimensions of illness experiences, health care-seeking processes and preferences, and practitioner-patient interactions;
- How often users of CAM, including patients and providers, adhere to treatment instructions and guidelines;
- The effects of CAM on wellness and disease-prevention;
- How the American public accesses and evaluates information about CAM modalities;
- Adverse events associated with CAM therapies and interactions between CAM and conventional treatments.

Further, the committee recommends that the National Library of Medicine and other federal agencies develop criteria to assess the quality and reliability of information about CAM.

We are in the midst of an exciting time of discovery, when evidence-based approaches to health bring opportunities for incorporating the best from all sources of care, be they conventional medicine or CAM. Our challenge is to keep an open mind and to regard each treatment possibility with an appropriate degree of skepticism. Only then will we be able to ensure that we are making informed and reasoned decisions.

1

Introduction

The widespread use of complementary and alternative medicine (CAM) is of major importance to today's health care consumers, practitioners, researchers, and policy makers. For example, look at the following statistics on CAM: 42 percent of people in the United States report that they have used at least one CAM therapy: however, less than 40 percent of those using CAM disclosed such use to a physician. In 1997, an estimated 15 million adults took prescription medications concurrently with herbal remedies or high-dose vitamins, bringing into play the possibility of negative interactions. Total visits to CAM providers exceed total visits to all primary-care physicians. Out-of-pocket costs for CAM are estimated to exceed $27 billion, which shows that CAM is now big business. Hospitals, managed care plans, and conventional practitioners are incorporating CAM therapies into their practices. Medical schools, nursing schools, and schools of pharmacy are teaching their students about CAM. Information about CAM flows freely in various media: newspapers, magazines, books, pamphlets, and the Internet. Friends talk to friends about remedies for specific problems.

Just what is CAM? Who is using CAM, and why are they doing so? Are CAM therapies safe? Are they effective? These are just a few of the questions surrounding the use of CAM by the American public. This chapter provides a framework for thinking about questions related to CAM use, explores the definition of CAM, describes a taxonomy for thinking about various CAM modalities, provides an overview of recent events in the history of CAM use in the United States, and briefly describes CAM activities currently under way at the National Institutes of Health (NIH) and the Agency for Healthcare Research and Quality (AHRQ).

This chapter begins by setting the context for the committee's consideration of CAM on the basis of a more general model of health care decision making.

CONTEXT

Questions about CAM use arise at a time when providers of conventional medical care are being challenged as never before to examine the effectiveness and efficiency of health care in the United States. The Institute of Medicine's (IOM's) *Crossing the Quality Chasm* (IOM, 2001) provides ample evidence for the underuse of effective care, the overuse of marginally effective or ineffective care, and the misuse of care, including preventable errors, in its delivery. Widespread variation in rates of surgery and other interventions for common conditions among seemingly similar populations in different geographic regions raises concern about how doctors and patients make decisions.

The *Crossing the Quality Chasm* report concludes that fragmentary, incremental change will be insufficient to reach achievable levels of quality improvement in American health care. Fundamental redesign will be required, and the report offers 10 rules for redesign. Taken together, these suggestions advocate a systems-minded approach to making health care more knowledge based and patient centered.

This report is about CAM, not about the quality of conventional medicine or the way in which it is delivered. However, as will be seen, central to the definition of CAM is that its constituent elements are "other than" conventional medicine. Therefore, an appreciation of both the strengths and the limitations of conventional medicine, especially as perceived by CAM users in the United States, is necessary context for development of conceptual models to guide public and private decision making about CAM research and practices.

The principal conceptual model that the committee used to frame this report begins with the question, What do patients and health professionals need to know to make good decisions about the use of health care interventions, including CAM? Corollary questions for policy makers relate to the research necessary to support decisions as well as policies and resources to ensure the quality and efficiency of services as well as equitable access. The more general nature of the question and its corollaries, addressing health care interventions rather than CAM interventions alone, reflects the committee's view that the decision-making needs of stakeholders in the American health care economy are equivalent for conventional and CAM health care services.

For the patient with symptoms or signs that diminish the quality of life or raise concerns about the length of life, answers to simple but compelling questions are necessary for decision making. What is wrong? What will happen if I do nothing: will things get better, worse, or stay the same? What are my treatment options, and what are the benefits and harms? What will the experience of treatment feel like? How likely am I to benefit, by how much, and for how long? How likely am I to be harmed, in what way, and for how long? Those who are well and want to stay that way by preventing preventable illness ask similar questions. The best answers to these questions come from a professional knowledge base that may be more or less supported by conclusive evidence relevant to the circumstances of the particular patient at hand. When such evidence does exist and is effectively marshaled and communicated, the decisions and resulting care attain the goal of being "knowledge based."

Good decisions depend on more than professional knowledge about treatment options and probabilities of outcomes. Different patients may be more or less bothered by the same symptoms. They may react differently to the experience of treatment itself and anticipate different reactions to the benefits or the harms, or both. Furthermore, no matter how good the evidence, there is always some uncertainty about outcomes for the individual patient. Risks that are acceptable to some may be unacceptable to others. Benefits or harms may be more or less likely to occur early or late, and patients' willingness to make trade-offs between the two is variably influenced by the timing of the good versus the bad. When particular patients' attitudes and preferences are elicited and respected, decisions about treatment and prevention and the resulting care attain the goal of being "patient centered."

It has been argued that there is much unwarranted variation in medical practice because of failures related to management of the professional knowledge base. In some cases the necessary research has not been done. In others, it is inaccessible to clinicians at the time that decisions are made. Evidence is also misinterpreted or inappropriately applied to a patient who is different from those whose experience provided the basis for the evidence. Furthermore, different clinicians have different understandings of how a profession knows what it knows and how the knowledge base is advanced. These epistemological differences may be even greater among users of conventional and CAM interventions.

Among clinicians who practice conventional medicine, there has been a marked shift over past decades from a reliance on professional experience to a greater emphasis on more rigorous quantitative evidence derived from randomized trials and systematic reviews of multiple trials. These more rigorous approaches have more recently been used in investigations of CAM. However, among the heterogeneous interventions that comprise CAM, particularly those that depend on variable practitioner approaches and the customization of interventions to individual patients, there are significant obstacles to use of the methods that have gained dominance in testing and advancing the knowledge base for conventional medical practitioners.

Despite the evident differences between conventional clinical practice and CAM, perhaps the most promising way to find common ground is to ask the question, What kind of knowledge do people need to make good health care decisions, and how can that knowledge be continuously tested and improved? This question provides the framework for considering the appropriate clinical and policy responses to the widespread use of CAM by the American public.

Furthermore, this framework is based on a set of ethical commitments that informed the work of the committee as it proceeded with its task. These commitments are explored in detail in Chapter 6:

1. a social commitment to public welfare,
2. a commitment to protect patients and the public,
3. respect for patient autonomy,
4. a recognition of medical pluralism, and
5. public accountability.

One of the first questions that the committee considered was, What is CAM? The following section explores this issue.

DEFINITION OF CAM

One of the difficulties in any study of CAM is trying to determine what is included in the definition of CAM. Does CAM include vitamin use, nutrition and diets, behavioral medicine, exercise and other treatments that have been integrated into conventional medical systems? Should CAM include prayer, shamanism, or other therapies that may not be considered health care practices? As discussed further in Chapter 6, the reasons for defining modalities as "CAM therapies" are not only scientific but also "political, social, [and] conceptual" (Jonas, 2002). In the United States, some of the most frequently used and well-known therapies that are recognized as CAM are relaxation techniques, herbs, chiropractic, and massage therapy (Eisenberg et al., 1998). Chiropractic, acupuncture, and massage therapy are licensed in most states. Naturopathy and homeopathy are licensed in fewer states. Numerous other therapies and modalities are considered unlicensed practices and at present few or no formal regulations apply to these therapies and modalities. The New York State Office of Regulatory Reform and CAM has identified more than 100 therapies, practices, and systems that could be considered CAM (see Appendix A for a list of therapies).

A lack of consistency in the definition of what is included in CAM is found throughout the literature. The National Center for Complementary and Alternative Medicine (NCCAM) of NIH defines CAM as "a group of diverse medical and health care systems, practices, and products that are not presently considered to be part of conventional medicine" (NCCAM, 2002). However, many would argue that a therapy does not cease to be a CAM therapy because it has been proven to be safe and effective and is used in conventional practice. "Simply because an herbal remedy comes to be used by physicians does not mean that herbalists cease to practice, or that the practice of the one becomes like that of the other" (Hufford, 2002:29).

Descriptive definitions of CAM include one by Ernst et al. (1995), who write that CAM is a "diagnosis, treatment and/or prevention which complements mainstream medicine by contributing to a common whole, satisfying a demand not met by orthodox, or diversifying the conceptual framework of medicine." Gevitz (1988) proposes that CAM includes "practices that are not accepted as correct, proper, or appropriate or are not in conformity with the beliefs or standards of the dominant group of medical practitioners in a society." In 1993, Eisenberg et al. defined CAM as "interventions neither taught widely in medical schools nor generally available in hospitals."

Kopelman (2002) argues that descriptive definitions such as those offered by Ernst et al. and Gevitz do not adequately answer the question, What is CAM? Definitions that place CAM outside the politically dominant health care system fail "to offer a standard for differentiating conventional interventions and CAM other than by appealing to what is or is not intrinsic to the practices of the dominant culture. This assumes there is a reliable and useful way to count cultures or subcultures and sort them into those that are dominant and those that are not" (Kopelman, 2002). Other descriptive definitions fail because conditions change, and therefore, descriptions of the conditions are no longer accurate. For example, look at the definition of Eisenberg and colleagues (1993), which states that CAM comprises inteventions that are neither taught widely in medical schools nor generally available in hospitals; however, more than half of all U.S. medical schools provide education about CAM, health care institutions are offering CAM services, and the numbers of insurers offering reimbursement for CAM therapies is growing (see Chapters 7 and 8).

According to Kopelman, normative definitions (e.g., untested or unscientific) also fail to distinguish CAM from conventional medicine. For example, Angell and Kassier (1998) write "there is only medicine that has been adequately tested and medicine that has not." However such a definition does not distinguish between conventional medicine and CAM because many conventional treatments have not been supported by rigorous testing. For example, a review of 160 Cochrane systematic reviews of the effectiveness of conventional biomedical procedures found that 20 percent showed no effect, whereas insufficient evidence was available for another 21 percent (Ezzo et al., 2001). Furthermore, "some CAM manufacturers adopt higher standards than are currently required in the United States and rigorously test their CAM products" (Kopelman, 2002).

Stipulative definitions (i.e., lists of therapies) are not successful in distinguishing CAM from conventional therapies, Kopelman argues, because they are not consistent from source to source and they provide no justification for the exclusion of therapies that are not included.

Given the lack of a consistent definition of CAM, some have tried to bring clarity to the situation by proposing classification systems that can be used to organize the field. One of the most widely used classification structures, developed by NCCAM (2000), divides CAM modalities into five categories:

1. Alternative medical systems,
2. Mind-body interventions,
3. Biologically based treatments,
4. Manipulative and body-based methods, and
5. Energy therapies.

As the name implies, alternative medical systems is a category that extends beyond a single modality, and refers to an entire system of theory and practice that developed separately from conventional medicine. Examples of these systems include traditional Chinese medicine, ayurvedic medicine, homeopathy, and naturopathy.

The second category in the NCCAM classification scheme is mind-body interventions, which include practices that are based on the human mind, but that have an effect on the human body and physical health, such as meditation, prayer, and mental healing.

The third category, biologically based therapies, includes specialized diets, herbal products, and other natural products such as minerals, hormones, and biologicals. Specialized diets include those proposed by Drs. Atkins and Ornish, as well as the broader field of functional foods that may reduce the risk of disease or promote health. A few of the well-known herbals for which there is evidence of effectiveness include St. John's wort for the treatment of mild to moderate depression and *Ginkgo biloba* for the treatment of mild cognitive impairment. An example of a nonherbal natural product is fish oil for the treatment of cardiovascular conditions.

The fourth category, manipulative and body-based methods, includes therapies that involve movement or manipulation of the body. Chiropractic is the best known in this category, and chiropractors are licensed to practice in every U.S. state. A defining feature of chiropractic treatment is spinal manipulation, also known as spinal adjustment, to correct spinal joint abnormalities (Meeker and Haldeman, 2002). Massage therapy is another example of a body-based therapy.

The final category described by NCCAM is energy therapies which include the manipulation and application of energy fields to the body. In addition to electromagnetic fields outside of the body, it is hypothesized that energy fields exist within the body. The existence of these biofields has not been experimentally proven; however, a number of therapies include them, such as qi gong, Reiki, and therapeutic touch.

A different approach to classifying CAM modalities is a descriptive taxonomy that groups therapies according to their philosophical and theoretical identities (Kaptchuk and Eisenberg, 2001). Practices are divided into two groups. The first group appeals to the general public and has become popularly known as CAM. This group includes professionalized or distinct medical systems (e.g., chiropratic, acupuncture, homeopathy), popular health reform (e.g., dietary supplement use and specialized diets), New Age healing (e.g., qi gong, Reiki, magnets), psychological interventions, and nonnormative scientific enterprises (conventional therapies used in unconventional ways or unconventional therapies used by conventionally trained medical or scientific professionals). The second group includes practices that are more relevant to specific populations, such as ethnic or religious groups (e.g., Native American traditional medicine, Puerto Rican spiritis, folk medicine, and religious healing).

This discussion of definitions shows that no clear and consistent definition of CAM exists, nor is there a recognized taxonomy to organize the field, although the one proposed by NCCAM is commonly used. Given the committee's charge and focus, for the purposes of this report, the committee has chosen to use as its working definition of CAM a modification of the definition proposed by the Panel on Definition and Description at a 1995 NIH research methodology conference (Defining and describing complementary and alternative medicine, 1997). This modified definition states that

> Complementary and alternative medicine (CAM) is a broad domain of resources that encompasses health systems, modalities, and practices and their accompanying theories and beliefs, other than those intrinsic to the dominant health system of a particular society or culture in a given historical period. CAM includes such resources perceived by their users as associated with positive health outcomes. Boundaries within CAM and between the CAM domain and the domain of the dominant system are not always sharp or fixed.

The committee chose this definition for several reasons. First, this broad definition reflects the scope and essence of CAM as used by the American public. Second, it avoids excluding common practices from the research agenda. The effect of such a broad definition means that all statements and recommendations made in this report will not apply equally to all CAM modalities and there may even be some CAM modalities for which particular statements do not apply at all. The third reason for choosing to define CAM as stated above is that it is patient centered and includes practices that people perceive to have health benefits. Fourth, it encompasses the potential for change. That is, this definition allows a therapy to be accepted as standard practice when there is evidence of effectiveness but still allows the therapy to remain a part of CAM. Furthermore, the chosen definition recognizes that the definition of "conventional" medicine will vary from time to time and from country to country, it does not presume that proven practices will be adopted, and it allows CAM to be evaluated over time.

The next section of this chapter is devoted to describing milestones in the recent history of CAM in the United States.

RECENT MILESTONES IN THE HISTORY OF CAM

In 1992 the U.S. Congress established the Office of Unconventional Therapies, later changed to the Office of Alternative Medicine (OAM), to explore "unconventional medical practices." Two million dollars was appropriated, and OAM began to develop a baseline of information on CAM use in the United States. *Alternative Medicine: Expanding Medical Horizons* was released in 1995 (Workshop on Alternative Medicine, 1995) and summarized the results of two workshops on CAM convened by OAM. The report (often referred to as the "Chantilly Report" because the workshops were held in Chantilly, Virginia, in 1992) examined six fields of alternative medicine and addressed issues such as research infrastructure, research databases, and research methodologies. Many of the recommendations made addressed research needs and opportunities. The report was significant because it was the result of the first NIH-sanctioned meetings held to discuss the field of CAM as a whole.

Responding to public and industry input, Congress passed the Dietary Supplement Health and Education Act (DSHEA) in 1994. DSHEA legally established the term "dietary supplement" and decreed that supplements were to be regulated similar to foods. This distinction exempted manufacturers from conducting premarketing safety and efficacy testing and eliminated the Food and Drug Administrations's (FDA's) premarketing regulatory authority. In 1995, NIH funded the Research Centers Program to provide a nationwide focus for interdisciplinary CAM research in academic institutions. Also in 1995, following a 1994 NIH and FDA workshop on acupuncture, FDA declassified acupuncture needles as an experimental product. In 1996 the Public Information Clearinghouse on CAM was established and NIH sponsored the Consensus Conference on Acupuncture, which provided evidence of the effectiveness of acupuncture for some conditions (e.g., dental pain and nausea).

The first large, multicenter trial of a CAM therapy was cofunded in 1997 by OAM, the National Institute on Mental Health, and the NIH Office of Dietary Supplements. The trial tested the effect of *Hypericum* (St. John's wort) for depression.

By 1998 the use of CAM was widely discussed and hotly debated. A *New England Journal of Medicine* editorial (Angell and Kassirer, 1998) argued that "It's time for the scientific community to stop giving CAM a free ride. There can not be two kinds of medicine—conventional and alternative. There is only medicine that has been adequately tested and medicine that has not, medicine that works and medicine that may or may not work." An editorial in the *Journal of the American Medical Association* contended that "There is no Alternative Medicine. There is only scientifically proven, evidence-based medicine supported by solid data or unproven medicine, for which scientific evidence is lacking" (Fontanarosa and Lundberg, 1998). The American Medical Association devoted space to the topic of CAM in its theme journals and published a total of 80 articles and the results of 18 randomized trials. Included were editorials, descriptive articles, systematic reviews, and results of randomized controlled trials. For the first time, CAM was addressed as a complex issue and journal editors were willing to subject these articles to the same criteria and editorial review as articles addressing topics in conventional medicine.

Meanwhile, Congress, having increased the OAM budget from the original $2 million to $19.5 million, elevated OAM to the level of a national center named NCCAM in 1998, awarded it $48.9 million for fiscal year (FY) 1999, and required that NCCAM appoint CAM practitioners as members of its Advisory Council. In 1999, the Cancer Advisory Panel for CAM was established for the purpose of assessing clinical data related to CAM treatment of cancer and the first Dietary Supplements Research Center was funded jointly by NCCAM and the NIH Office of Dietary Supplements. NIH funded nine Centers for Research of Complementary and Alternative Medicine to conduct interdisciplinary research and training. Three multicenter research studies were funded: one on *Ginkgo biloba* for the treatment of dementia (cofunded by NCCAM and the National Institute on Aging), one on glucosamine and chondroitin sulfate for the treatment of knee osteoarthritis (cofunded by NCCAM and the National Institute of Arthritis and Musculoskeletal and Skin Diseases), and one on acupuncture for osteoarthritis of the knee (funded by NCCAM). Also in 1999 large pharmaceutical companies entered the CAM market with herbal product lines and other dietary supplements.

Several major events occurred in 2000 and 2001. In March 2000, President Clinton created the White House Commission on Complementary and Alternative Medicine Policy. The purpose of the commission was to "study and report on public policy issues in the rapidly expanding field of complementary and alternative medicine." Furthermore, the commission was asked to report on "legislative and administrative recommendations to assure that public policy maximizes the benefits to Americans of appropriate use of complementary and alternative medicine" (Executive Order 13147, 2000). The commission's report provided recommendations about research on CAM, education and training in CAM, CAM information dissemination, delivery of CAM practices, coverage and reimbursement for CAM services, the potential role of CAM in wellness and health promotion, and the need for coordination of CAM-related efforts (WHCCAMP, 2002).

The Federation of State Medical Boards began work on CAM guidelines for physicians in 2000. The initiative was focused on "encouraging the medical community to adopt consistent standards, ensuring the public health and safety by facilitating the proper and effective use of both conventional and CAM treatments, while educating physicians on the adequate safeguards needed to assure these services are provided within the bounds of acceptable professional practice" (FSMB, 2002). The federation's House of Delegates approved the guidelines in April 2002.

The Consortium of Academic Health Centers for Integrative Medicine was launched in 2000 and by 2003 it had 22 member medical schools (see Appendix B for a list of member centers). To become a member, either the dean or chancellor is required to commit to developing programs in research, education, and clinical delivery of CAM and the school must demonstrate an organized and robust program in two of those three areas. The mission of the consortium is "to help transform medicine and healthcare through rigorous scientific studies, new models of clinical care, and innovative educational programs that integrate biomedicine, the complexity of human beings, the intrinsic nature of healing and the rich diversity of therapeutic systems" (Consortium of Academic Health Centers for Integrative Medicine, 2004).

Skeptics of CAM had long contended that the only benefit derived from CAM therapies was due to a placebo effect, not "real" effects. In November 2000 NIH hosted a workshop, The Science of the Placebo: Toward an Interdisciplinary Research Agenda, thereby helping to place placebo in the category of a "real" effect. The August 2001 issue of *Science* published an article on basic science mechanisms of placebo (de la Fuente-Fernandez et al., 2001). These two events triggered expanded interest among the neuroscience community in the study of the impact of nonspecific effects (e.g., expectation, context, belief) on clinical outcomes. Placebo was no longer something to be discarded or dismissed but, rather, something to be studied.

Also in 2001, NCCAM and the National Library of Medicine developed CAM on PubMed, a free, web-based access to journal citations directly related to CAM. At present, almost 40,000 citations on CAM can be found on the PubMed website. Additionally, clinically significant adverse drug-herb interactions were documented in case studies (Fugh-Berman, 2000), and St. John's wort was shown to reduce the level of indinavir, a protease inhibitor taken by AIDS patients, in plasma (Piscitelli et al., 2000).

In 2002, NCCAM launched its Intramural Program to explore CAM treatment strategies for patients at the NIH Clinical Center, the world's largest facility dedicated to patient-oriented research. Also in that year, the U.S. Department of Veterans Affairs agreed to provide reimbursement for chiropractic care, the *Annals of Internal Medicine* began a special series on CAM (17 publications), and *Science Xpress* published an article on positron emission spectrometry, imaging of the placebo response versus the response to opiod analgesics, thereby signalling continued interest in the application of modern technology to the mechanistic study of placebo-related phenomena.

NCCAM, whose budget had grown to $104.6 million in 2002, funded 10 international planning grants, and across NIH more than 200 research projects on CAM were ongoing. Also in that year, IOM established the Committee on the Use of Complementary and Alternative Medicine by the American Public. In 2003, the first two Centers of Excellence for Research on CAM were funded to increase scientific rigor in research on CAM. By 2004 the NCCAM budget was $117.8 million.

The following section explores in greater detail, the kinds of research and training efforts undertaken by NIH and the AHRQ

CAM ACTIVITIES AT NIH AND AHRQ

National Center for Complementary and Alternative Medicine

Twenty institutes and centers within NIH support ongoing CAM-related research, with NCCAM being the primary center for such research. According to the legislation creating NCCAM (P.L. 105-277), NCCAM's mandate is the "conduct and support of basic and applied research (intramural and extramural), research training, and [to] disseminate health information and other programs with respect to identifying, investigating, and validating CAM treatments, diagnostic and prevention modalities, disciplines and systems." To achieve its mandate, NCCAM focuses on four primary areas: research, research training and career development, outreach, and integration.

To guide its research efforts, NCCAM develops program priorities through a semiannual formal review process. At present, its three priority areas are to elucidate the mechanisms of action and conduct small, well-developed Phase I and II studies; build infrastructure to support research at CAM institutions; and encourage collaboration between institutions that provide conventional medical therapies and those that provide CAM therapies (http://nccam.nih.gov/research/priorities/index.htm).

The development of research centers is the main method used to pursue research. NCCAM's CAM-related research centers can be placed into several categories: Dietary Supplement Research, Developmental Centers that partner institutions where CAM is practiced and those where conventional medicine is practiced, Centers of Excellence, Centers for CAM Research, and Exploratory Program Grants for Frontier Medicine Research. The establishment of international centers for CAM research is also an initiative in development. Unlike the other centers at NIH, which invest about two-thirds of their research funding in basic research, NCCAM places the largest proportion of its resources in clinical research; the ratio of funding for clinical research to funding for basic research was 2.5:1 in FY 2003 (NCCAM, 2004).

An impressive number of patients are participating in NCCAM-supported clinical trials (10,708 participants in 2002), more than half of whom are in Phase III clinical trials. Research on prevention (e.g., research directed to such areas as dementia, prostate cancer, and myocardial infarction) is another emphasis of NCCAM, as are studies on women's health (e.g., research examining the effects of plant-based estrogens), research on reducing or eliminating health disparities, and age-related health research.

In addition to increasing support for research project grants and research centers, since FY 1999 NCCAM has dramatically increased the funding devoted to training, career, and curriculum awards (Straus, 2003). Such funds are consistent with NCCAM's goal of increasing the number of skilled CAM researchers by making awards for CAM-related research available to pre- and postdoctoral students, CAM practitioners, conventional medical researchers and practitioners, and members of underrepresented populations in scientific research (http://nccam.nih.gov/training/overview.htm).

NCCAM also participates in a variety of outreach efforts. It maintains several outlets for both the public and the research community. The NCCAM website (http://nccam.nih.gov/) provides detailed descriptions of its ongoing activities as well as fact sheets about CAM, information on factors related to decision making about treatments, cost and payment questions, and safety alerts and advisories. NCCAM also publishes a quarterly newsletter containing updates on new and ongoing activities of the center. NCCAM also uses lectures, town meetings, and exhibits at scientific meetings as opportunities to increase people's awareness of CAM and the center.

In addition, NCCAM has established a clearinghouse, accessible by Internet and telephone in both English and Spanish, for people seeking information about CAM. The clearinghouse does not provide medical advice but does disseminate scientifically based information on CAM. Two other activities that assist with outreach are publications in peer-reviewed scientific journals, the number of which is increasing, and the development of the *CAM on PubMed* subsection of the National Library of Medicine's MEDLINE database.

One of NCCAM's stated goals is to "integrate scientifically proven CAM practices into conventional medicine" (http://nccam.nih.gov/about/aboutnccam/index.htm). Integration is an obvious extension of NCCAM's investments in research, research training, and expanding outreach. NCCAM hopes to aid integration by publishing research results, investigating ways in which evidence-based CAM practices can be integrated into conventional medical practice, and supporting programs that develop models for the incorporation of CAM into medical, dental, and nursing school curricula.

NCCAM is in the process of developing its second 5-year strategic plan, which will be released in January 2005. NCCAM plans to continue focusing on research, research training, outreach, and integration and intends for its second strategic plan to provide greater specificity and prioritization within these areas.

One can see from this discussion that NCCAM has an impressive and well-organized series of activities designed to advance the state of knowledge about CAM therapies and their use. NCCAM's mandated focus is on CAM, however other centers and institutes within the NIH also have impressive portfolios evaluating CAM therapies. NCCAM established the 40-member Trans-Agency CAM Coordinating Committee in 1999 to foster collaboration across these various institutes and other federal agencies involved with research on CAM. The following section describes some of the activities of NIH institutes and centers.

NIH Institutes and Centers

As seen in Table 1-1, institutes and centers other than NCCAM collectively spend millions of dollars on CAM-related activities. The NIH institutes and centers conduct research in partnership with each other and independently, facilitating a broad scope of activity in both clinical and basic research. There is ongoing research on the safety and efficacy of CAM practices for disease treatment and prevention; mechanisms of therapies including dietary supplements such as soy isoflavones and acupuncture; placebo effects; the role of spirituality in health; as well as animal studies of alternative therapies for Parkinson's disease. Table 1-1 displays the level of funding for CAM research by center or institute for the past few years.

TABLE 1-1 CAM Funding by NIH Institute or Center

Participating Institutes and Centers[a]	1997	1998	1999	2000
NCI	2.2	28.2	36.6	43.0
NHLBI	5.9	5.6	2.8	4.1
NIDCR	0.2	0.3	0.3	0.6
NIDDK	1.2	1.2	1.4	1.6
NINDS	4.3	5.8	5.3	4.6
NIAID	3.4	6.2	7.5	7.9
NICHD	1.2	0.4	1.2	1.6
NEI	0.7	0.8	0.7	1.0
NIEHS	1.2	2.9	1.4	3.0
NIA	2.8	3.3	3.1	6.0
NIAMS	0.2	2.2	0.2	0.3
NIMH	2.7	3.8	5.1	5.8
NIDA	0.4	0.3	0.4	0.3
NIAAA	0.3	0.3	0.0	1.1
NINR	0.6	0.7	1.7	3.3
NCRR	2.9	5.5	6.8	7.4
NCCAM	—	0.0	40.5	77.8
NCMHD	—	—	—	—
FIC	0.6	0.6	0.6	0.6
OD	10.6	19.5	0.0	0.1
NIH	42.0	88.0	116.0	170.6

NOTE: Amounts are in millions of dollars per fiscal year. Note that various institutes may use different definitions of CAM.

[a]See Appendix C for full names of centers.

Office of Cancer Complementary and Alternative Medicine

The Office of Cancer Complementary and Alternative Medicine (OCCAM) within the National Cancer Institute (NCI) develops and coordinates CAM activities related to cancer. OCCAM was established in 1998. Program efforts are divided among three areas: Research Development and Support Program, Practice Assessment Program, and Communications Program.

The Research Development and Support Program funds research on CAM for the prevention, diagnosis, and treatment of cancer; CAM for cancer-related symptoms; and CAM modalities that can address the side effects of conventional treatment. Examples of recent activities include a methodology working group on research on cancer symptom management by the use of CAM, the provision of competitive supplementary funds for

2001	2002	2003	2004 Estimate	2005 Estimate
50.8	85.3	123.5	128.5	132.4
6.2	8.9	7.2	7.4	7.5
0.9	0.9	0.8	0.8	0.8
1.8	2.4	3.2	3.3	3.4
6.6	6.8	4.5	4.6	4.7
8.0	11.5	18.8	19.2	19.4
3.1	2.5	1.7	1.7	1.8
1.0	2.1	2.8	2.9	3.0
3.2	3.6	4.9	5.0	5.2
5.1	5.2	7.1	7.3	7.5
0.6	1.6	1.7	1.7	1.8
6.7	3.9	5.9	6.1	6.3
0.3	0.3	1.2	1.2	1.3
1.3	1.7	1.5	1.5	1.5
4.2	4.1	3.1	3.2	3.2
6.1	6.6	7.7	7.8	8.1
89.1	104.3	113.4	116.9	121.1
—	0.2	0.2	0.2	0.2
0.6	0.7	0.8	0.8	0.8
16.7	0.2	5.6	4.8	4.9
212.9	252.9	315.5	325.0	334.9

SOURCE: NIH Office of the Director, Office of Budget, Budget Reporting and Legislative Branch. Available at: http://nccam.nih.gov/about/budget/institute-center.htm [accessed March 31, 2004].

NCI-designated cancer centers, and a workshop on how to write a grant to receive funding for research on cancer-related CAM modalities.

The Practice Assessment Program has two primary objectives: (1) to evaluate potential therapies and assess whether future research is warranted and (2) to build a dialogue between health practitioners and researchers about CAM and cancer issues. The Practice Assessment supports the Best Case Series Program for groups of cancer patients treated with CAM therapies. Examples of best case series that have been completed are the Kelly-Gonzalez Regimen for pancreatic cancer and insulin potentiation therapy investigated by Steven Ayre.

Lastly, the Communications Program develops and disseminates information about NCI activities and obtains feedback about interests and obstacles in CAM-related research on cancer. Like NCCAM, OCCAM sponsors conferences, lectures, and expert panels to increase the quality and awareness of ongoing CAM-related research on cancer.

Office of Dietary Supplements

The Office of Dietary Supplements (ODS) is part of the Office of NIH Director and was established in 1995 in response to a congressional mandate (DSHEA, 1994). Its mission is to "strengthen knowledge and understanding of dietary supplements by evaluating scientific information, stimulating and supporting research, disseminating research results, and educating the public to foster an enhanced quality of life and health for the U.S. population."

ODS, unlike the NIH institutes and centers, cannot directly fund investigator-initiated research. However, it partners with the NIH institutes and centers and government and private agencies to achieve its mission by supporting research, sponsoring conferences, and disseminating information. In January 2004, ODS released its 2004-2009 Strategic Plan, its second such plan, which contained five overarching goals related to research, information communication, and education. Although these goals have been adopted for the second strategic plan, greater emphasis will be placed on the use of emerging technologies, cross-disciplinary studies, training and education of investigators, translation of research, and establishment of a process for regular evaluation of ODS programs and activities.

In the last 5 years, ODS has initiated many efforts to improve the quality of research on dietary supplements. For example, ODS established a program to enhance analytical methodologies and develop standard reference preparations of dietary supplements and also created two databases that are accessible to everyone: the Computer Access to Research on Dietary Supplements database (CARDS) and the International Bibliographic Information on Dietary Supplements (IBIDS). CARDS contains information on federally funded dietary supplement research and is continually updated. IBIDS provides access to bibliographic citations and abstracts from published, international, scientific literature on dietary supplements. An additional resource for the research community and general public are evidence-based review reports commissioned through a partnership between ODS and NCCAM from AHRQ Evidence-Based Practice Centers.

ODS, in various partnerships with NCCAM, the National Institute for Environmental Health Sciences, the Office of Research on Women's Health, and the National Institute of General Medical Sciences, funds six Centers for Dietary Supplement Research. The centers emphasize botanicals and aim to identify and characterize these compounds, assess their bioavailabilities and activities, explore their mechanisms of action, conduct preclinical and clinical evaluations, establish training and career development, and help select the botanicals to be tested in clinical trials.

Agency for Healthcare Research and Quality

The AHRQ, which is part of the U.S. Department of Health and Human Services, is authorized to sponsor, conduct, and disseminate research to improve the quality and effectiveness of health care. AHRQ administers Evidence-Based Practice Centers (EPCs), which have produced evidence-based reports requested by other federal agencies on the effectiveness and safety of a limited number of dietary supplements. The reports of the EPCs are based on a systematic analysis of the relevant scientific data and are designed to differentiate the types and strengths of a comprehensive body of evidence.

Nominations for clinical topics to be reviewed by an EPC are solicited through notices in the *Federal Register*. The clinical topics must meet specific selection criteria including a high incidence; significance for the needs of Medicare, Medicaid, or other federal health programs; high cost; controversy about their effectiveness; and the availability of scientific data. On the basis of this process, reports on six dietary supplements[1] have been reviewed as of October 2003. In addition to the evidence-based practice reports, AHRQ also funds investigator-initiated research and supports a small number of grants for CAM-related research.

The Institute of Medicine Study of CAM

The previous pages have described the progress that has been made in evaluating and understanding CAM. Yet, numerous challenges remain to be confronted as individuals seek to make decisions about the safety, effectiveness, and use of various CAM therapies and modalities. In September 2002, NCCAM, 15 other NIH centers and institutes, and AHRQ commissioned the IOM to conduct a study on the use of CAM by the American public. Specifically, the study was to:

1. Describe the use of CAM therapies by the American public and provide a comprehensive overview, to the extent that data are available, of the therapies in widespread use, the populations that use them, and what is known about how they are provided.

---

[1]The topics of the six reports are as follows: Antioxidant supplements for the prevention and treatment of cancer (October 2003); Antioxidant supplements for the prevention and treatment of cardiovascular disease (CVD) (July 2003); Ephedra and ephedrine for weight loss and athletic performance enhancement (March 2003); S-adenosyl-L-Methionine (SAMe) for depression, osteoarthritis, and liver disease (August 2002); Garlic for CVD cardiovascular disease (October 2000); and Milk thistle effects (September 2000).

2. Identify major scientific, policy, and practice issues related to CAM research and to the translation of validated therapies into conventional medical practice.

3. Develop conceptual models or frameworks to guide public- and private-sector decision making as research and practice communities confront the challenges of conducting research on CAM, translating research findings into practice, and addressing the distinct policy and practice barriers inherent in that translation.

Guidance was specifically sought on the following matters:

• Study the methodological difficulties in the conduct of rigorous research on CAM therapies and how these relate to issues in regulation and practice, with exploration of options to address the identified difficulties.

• The shortage of highly skilled practitioners who are able to participate in scientific inquiry that meets NIH guidelines and who have access to the institutions where such research is conducted.

• The shortage of receptive, integrated research environments and the barriers to developing multidisciplinary teams that include CAM and conventional medical practitioners.

• The availability of standardized and well-characterized materials and practices to be studied and incorporated, when appropriate, into practice.

• Existing decision-making models used to determine whether or not to incorporate new therapies and practices into conventional medicine, including evidence thresholds.

• Applicability of these decision-making models to CAM therapies and practices; that is, do they form good precedents for decisions relating to regulation, accreditation, or integration of CAM therapies?

• Identification and analysis of successful approaches to the incorporation of CAM into health professions education.

• Impact of current regulation and legislation on CAM research and integration.

IOM convened the Committee on the Use of Complementary and Alternative Medicine (CAM) by the American Public. Between February 2003 and May 2004 the committee met seven times and held five information-gathering workshops, during which testimony was solicited from any individual wishing to provide input to the committee. Over the course of this study the committee met and talked with representatives of various federal agencies, the CAM and conventional medicine communities, researchers, practitioners, educators, and patients. A liaison panel was convened with representatives both from CAM practice communities and from the conventional medicine community (Appendix D). The liaison panel met with the committee three times and provided critical input regarding many important issues including major challenges, methodological issues (e.g., outcome concepts and measures), and factors facilitating or inhibiting communication and cooperation across disciplines.

Collectively, the committee read, summarized, and analyzed articles and other information on CAM therapies, evaluation of evidence, CAM-related decision making, education on CAM, and much more. The committee commissioned a paper on methodological issues, which provided the information from which Chapter 4 was developed. The work of the committee has been challenging yet rewarding. The results of that work are contained in this report.

REPORT CONTENTS

This report identifies the major scientific, policy, and practice issues related to CAM. It explores what is known about the use of CAM, the methods and approaches used for CAM-related research, and how this knowledge is being translated into practice. Finally, the report provides recommendations to research and practice communities as they make decisions and confront the challenges of conducting research on CAM, translate the research findings into practice, and address the distinct policy and practice barriers inherent in that translation.

This chapter has provided the context within which this report was developed, the definition and description of CAM, and a brief history and the present view of CAM-related activities under way at NIH and AHRQ. Chapter 2 describes what is known about the prevalence, cost, and patterns of use of CAM therapies and identifies the areas in which more information is needed. A discussion of the approaches to the evaluation of evidence of treatment effectiveness is presented in Chapter 3. Chapter 4 examines the need for innovative designs in research on CAM. Chapter 5 explores the existing evidence of the effectiveness for CAM and the gaps in that evidence and describes a research framework for use in filling the gaps that have been identified. Chapter 6 presents an ethical framework for CAM research, policy, and practice. Chapter 7 reviews the growing integration of CAM and explores why such integration is occurring, and Chapter 8 discusses the education of both conventional practitioners and CAM practitioners. Chapter 9 focuses on dietary supplements, and Chapter 10 presents the conclusion of the report.

For the body of the report, the committee reviewed a broad cross section of studies on use of CAM in clinical populations that were published in peer-reviewed journals. The list of studies was generated by a PubMed search covering the past 8 years plus all reviews of studies on

CAM use for particular health complaints and special populations. The committee did not seek to quantify such results as studies were carried out in different clinical settings using different procedures for data collection. CAM use in such settings was cited as common if such appeared to be the case or was cited as illustrative as noted in the text. Table 2-1 and much of the content for Chapter 2 relies on an exhaustive review of those epidemiological studies of CAM use by the U.S. public which involved random, nationally representative samples that were published in the peer-reviewed medical literature. Apart from those studies cited in Table 2-1, we are not aware of additional publications which meet these straightforward criteria.

For report comments in the qualitative realm (e.g., reasons why different types of people use CAM—Table 2-2) and those referring to individual populations (i.e., CAM use among population subgroups), publications were generated by (1) a PubMed search, (2) a search of major health social science journals covering the fields of anthropology, sociology, psychology and geography, and (3) a library search of books and book chapters on CAM written by those holding advanced academic degrees and having academic positions in reputable U.S., Canadian, Australian, and British universities. Data on the range of motivations for using CAM was qualitative, and the committee made no attempt to quantify results. Data on the lack of studies on compliance/adherence with CAM was based on a PubMed search that went back 12 years.

REFERENCES

Angell M, Kassirer JP. 1998. Alternative medicine—the risks of untested and unregulated remedies. *N Engl J Med* 339(12):839–841.

Consortium of Academic Health Centers for Integrative Medicine. 2004. [Online]. Available at: http://www.imconsortium.org/index.php. [accessed June 16, 2004].

Defining and describing complementary and alternative medicine. 1997. Panel on Definition and Description, CAM Research Methodology Conference, April 1995. *Altern Ther Health Med* 3(2):49–57.

de la Fuente-Fernandez R, Ruth TJ, Sossi V, Schulzer M, Calne DB, Stoessl AJ. 2001. Expectation and dopamine release: Mechanism of the placebo effect in Parkinson's disease. *Science* 293(5532):1164–1166.

DSHEA (Dietary Supplement Health and Education Act of 1994). Public Law No. 103-417, 108 Stat. 4325, 21 U.S.C. ss. 301 et seq. 1994.

Eisenberg DM, Kessler RC, Foster C, Norlock FE, Calkins DR, Delbanco TL. 1993. Unconventional medicine in the United States: Prevalence, costs, and patterns of use. *N Engl J Med* 328:246–252.

Eisenberg DM, Davis RB, Ettner SL, Appel S, Wilkey S, Van Rompay M, Kessler RC. 1998. Trends in alternative medicine use in the United States, 1990-1997: Results of a follow-up national survey. *JAMA* 280(18):1569–1575.

Ernst E, Resch KL, Mills S, Hill R, Mitchell A, Willoughby M, White A. 1995. Complementary medicine: A definition. *Br J Gen Pract* 45:506.

Executive Order 13147. 2000. White House Commission on Complementary and Alternative Medicine.

Ezzo J, Bausell B, Moerman DE, Berman B, Hadhazy V. 2001. Reviewing the reviews. How strong is the evidence? How clear are the conclusions? *Int J Technol Assess Health Care* 17(4):457–466.

Fontanarosa PB, Lundberg GD. 1998. Alternative medicine meets science. *JAMA* 280(18):1618–1619.

FSMB (Federation of State Medical Boards). 2002. *Model Guidelines for the Use of Complementary and Alternative Therapies in Medical Practice*. Dallas, TX: FSMB.

Fugh-Berman A. 2000. Herb-drug interactions. *Lancet* 355(9198):134–138.

Gevitz N. 1988. *Other Healers: Unorthodox Medicine in America*. Baltimore, MD: Johns Hopkins University Press.

Hufford DJ. 2002. CAM and Cultural Diversity: Ethics and Epistemology Converge. In: Callahan D, ed. *The Role of Complementary and Alternative Medicine: Accommodating Pluralism*.Washington DC: Georgetown University Press. Pp. 15–35.

IOM (Institute of Medicine). 2001. *Crossing the Quality Chasm: A New Health System for the 21st Century*. Washington DC: National Academy Press.

Jonas WB. 2002. Policy, the public, and priorities in alternative medicine research. *Ann Amer Acad Politi Soc Sci* 583:29–43.

Kaptchuk TJ, Eisenberg DM. 2001. Varieties of healing. 2: A taxonomy of unconventional healing practices. *Ann Intern Med* 135(3):196–204.

Kopelman LM. 2002. The Role of Science in Assessing Conventional, Complementary, and Alternative Medicines. In: Callahan D, ed. *The Role of Complementary and Alternative Medicine: Accommodating Pluralism*. Washington DC: Georgetown University Press. Pp. 36–53.

Meeker WC, Haldeman S. 2002. Chiropractic: A profession at the crossroads of mainstream and alternative medicine. *Ann Intern Med* 136(3):216–227.

NCCAM (National Center for Complementary and Alternative Medicine). 2000. *Expanding Horizons of Healthcare: Five-Year Strategic Plan 2001-2005*. NIH Publication No. 01-5001. Washington DC: U.S. Department of Health and Human Services.

NCCAM. 2002. *What Is Complementary and Alternative Medicine (CAM)?* [Online]. Available: http://nccam.nih.gov/health/whatiscam/index.htm [accessed June 10, 2004].

NCCAM. 2004. *National Center for Complementary and Alternative Medicine: The First Five Years*. Washington DC: DHHS.

NCI (National Cancer Institute). 2004. *The National Cancer Institute's Office of Complementary and Alternative Medicine*. Washington, DC: DHHS.

Piscitelli SC, Burstein AH, Chaitt D, Alfaro RM, Falloon J. 2000. Indinavir concentrations and St John's wort. *Lancet* 355(9203):547–548.

Straus S. 2003. NCCAM Research: Measures of success, lessons learned, and opportunities. Presentation given to the Committee on the Use of Complementary and Alternative Medicine by the American Public. Washington, DC: IOM.

WHCCAMP (White House Commission on Complementary and Alternative Medicine Policy). 2002. *Final Report*. Washington, DC: WHCCAMP.

Workshop on Alternative Medicine. 1995. *Alternative Medicine: Expanding Medical Horizons*. A Report to the National Institutes of Health on Alternative Medical Systems. Washington DC: NIH.

2

Prevalence, Cost, and Patterns of CAM Use

OVERALL USE

The first nationally representative survey of prevalence, costs, and patterns of use of complementary and alternative medicine (CAM) involved a random sample of 1,539 adults who were interviewed by phone in 1990. That survey inquired about the use of 16 CAM therapies and reported that one in three respondents (34 percent) had used at least one complementary therapy during the past year to treat their most serious or bothersome medical condition(s). It also found that those who saw providers for CAM therapies made an average of 19 visits per year, that complementary therapies were used primarily for chronic conditions as opposed to acute or life-threatening conditions, and that CAM therapies were predominantly used in addition to—and not as replacements for—conventional medical therapies. Importantly, it also found that 72 percent of CAM therapy users did not inform their medical doctors that they used CAM (Eisenberg et al., 1993).

Extrapolation of the results of the 1990 survey to the U.S. population suggests that in 1990 Americans made an estimated 425 million visits to providers of complementary care. This number exceeded the number of visits to U.S. primary care physicians (388 million) and was associated with an annual expenditure of approximately $13.7 billion, three-quarters of which ($10.3 billion) were paid out of pocket. This amount was comparable to the $12.8 billion spent out of pocket annually for all hospitalizations in the United States.

A national follow-up survey indicated a dramatic increase in CAM use by the American public between 1990 and 1997 (Eisenberg et al., 1998). (See Table 2-1 for a summary of the surveys of CAM use that have been conducted.) Specifically:

- The prevalence of CAM use increased by 25 percent from 33.8 percent in 1990 to 42.1 percent in 1997.
- The prevalence of herbal remedy use increased by 380 percent.
- The prevalence of high-dose vitamin use increased by 130 percent.
- The total number of visits to CAM providers increased by 47 percent from 427 million in 1990 to 629 million in 1997.
- The total visits to CAM providers (629 million) exceeded the total number of visits to all primary-care physicians (386 million) in 1997.
- It was estimated that, in 1997, adults made 33 million office visits to professionals for advice regarding the use of herbs and high-dose vitamins.
- An estimated 15 million adults in 1997 took prescription medications concurrently with herbal remedies or high-dose vitamins or both. These individuals are therefore at risk for potential adverse drug-herb or drug-supplement interactions.
- If insurance coverage for CAM therapies increases in the future, current use of CAM services is likely an under-representation of future utilization patterns.
- Despite the dramatic increases in the rates of use and the expenditures associated with CAM services, the extent to which patients disclosed their use of CAM therapies to their physicians remains low. In both 1990 and 1997, less than 40 percent of CAM therapy users disclosed to their physicians that they had used such therapies.
- Estimated expenditures for CAM professional services increased by 45 percent, exclusive of inflation. In 1997 such expenditures were estimated to be $21.2 billion.
- Out-of-pocket expenditures for herbal products and high-dose vitamins in 1997 were estimated to be $8.0 billion.
- Out-of-pocket expenditures for CAM professional services in 1997 were estimated to be $12.2 billion. This exceeded the out-of-pocket expenditures for all U.S. hospitalizations.
- Total out-of-pocket expenditures relating to CAM therapies were conservatively estimated to be $27.0 billion. This is comparable to the projected out-of-pocket expenditures for all U.S. physician services.

The study also found that among the respondents who in the past year had used CAM and seen their medical doctor, 63 to 72 percent did not disclose to their doctor the fact that they had received at least one type of CAM therapy. Among 507 respondents who reported their reasons for

TABLE 2-1 Use of Complementary/Alternative Medicine by U.S. Adults

Author (year)	Nature of Sample/Survey	Response Rate (%)	Description of Sample
Barnes et al. (2004)	Representative sample, n = 31,044, computer assisted personal interviews	74.3	Adults aged >18 years. Data were age adjusted to 2000 U.S. standard population
Ni et al. (2002)	Representative sample, n = 30,801, computer assisted personal interviews	70	Data from 1999 National Health Interview Survey. Adults aged >18 years. Data were age adjusted to 1999 U.S. population
Eisenberg et al. (1998)	Random, n = 2,055, telephone interview	60	Random sample of U.S. population 52% female 77% white

Questions Asked	Prevalence Figures by Therapy (%)
Questions were part of the 2002 National Health Interview Survey. Questions asked about use (ever and during past 12 months) of 27 types of CAM therapies (10 provider-based, and 17 non-provider based). If a CAM therapy was used in the last 12 months, respondents were also asked about: condition being treated; reason for choosing therapy, insurance coverage for costs; satisfaction with treatment; and whether conventional practitioner knew about CAM use.	Overall, in 2002, about 62% of U.S. adults used some form of CAM in the past 12 months. 10 CAM therapies most commonly used in past 12 months: 43.0% prayer for one's own health 24.4% prayer by other's for one's own health 18.9% natural products 11.6% deep breathing exercises 9.6% participation in prayer group for one's own health 7.6% meditation 7.5% chiropractic care 5.1% yoga 5.0% massage 3.5% diet-based therapies Medical Conditions: CAM most often used for back pain or problems, head or chest colds, neck pain or problems, joint pain or stiffness, and anxiety or depression.
Questions were part of the 1999 National Health Interview Survey. Participants were asked if, during the past 12 months, they had used any CAM therapies (from a list of 11).	28.9% of U.S. adults used at least one CAM therapy during the past year. Most commonly used therapies: 13.7% spiritual healing or prayer 9.6% herbal medicine 7.6% chiropractic therapies 6.9% lifestyle diet 6.4% massage therapy 5.0% relaxation 3.1% homeopathy 1.7% imagery 1.4% acupuncture 1.1% energy 0.5% hypnosis 0.5% biofeedback 0.3% other (e.g., qi gong, yoga, chelation, and bee stings)
Have you ever used any of the following forms of CAM (16 named) to treat your principle medical conditions? If so, have you done so within the last 12 months?	Used in the last 12 months: 42.0% at least one CAM 13.0% relaxation technique 12.0% herbal medicine 11.0% massage 11.0% chiropractic

continued

TABLE 2-1 Continued

Author (year)	Nature of Sample/Survey	Response Rate (%)	Description of Sample
Astin (1998)	Random sample of adults in the U.S., n = 1,035, representative of U.S. population	69	National Family Opinion Survey (USA) Age ≤ 18 51% female 80% white 30% high school or less 12% ≤12,500 annual income
Paramore (1997)	Representative, n = 3,450	75	Sample from the National Access to Care Survey
Eisenberg et al. (1993)	Representative, random, n = 1,539, telephone interview	67	Random sample from USA 48% female 34% aged > 50 years 32% white Sample recruited through random digit dialing

nondisclosure, common reasons were "It wasn't important for the doctor to know" (61 percent), "The doctor never asked" (60 percent), "It was none of the doctor's business" (31 percent), and "The doctor would not understand" (20 percent). Fewer respondents (14 percent) thought that their doctor would disapprove of or discourage CAM use, and just 2 percent thought that the doctor might not continue as their provider if the doctor knew that the patient had received some sort of CAM therapy. The respondents judged CAM therapies to be more helpful than conventional care for the treatment of headache and neck and back conditions, but they considered conventional care to be more helpful than CAM therapy for treatment of hypertension. Adults who use both CAM and conventional medicine appear to value both and tend to be less concerned about their medical doctors' disapproval than they are about their doctors' inability to understand or incorporate CAM therapy use within the context of their medical management (Eisenberg et al., 1998).

Paramore (1997) analyzed data from a national database composed of survey data for 3,450 individuals. The survey indicated that in 1994 approximately 10 percent of the adult population (25 million individuals) had seen a professional for at least one of four CAM therapies: chiropractic,

Questions Asked	Prevalence Figures by Therapy (%)

Have you used any of the following forms of CAM (17 named) within the past year?	40% has used CAM in the past year
	  16.0% chiropractic
	  8.0% lifestyle diet
	  7.0% exercise
	  7.0% relaxation

In the last year, did you see a professional for one of four therapies?	6.8% chiropractic 3.1% therapeutic massage 1.3% relaxation techniques 0.4% acupuncture

Have you ever used any of the following therapies (16 named) to treat your principle medical conditions? If so, have you done so within the last 12 months?	Used in the last 12 months:
	  34.0% at least one CAM
	  13.0% relaxation techniques
	  10.0% chiropractic
	  7.0% massage

relaxation techniques, therapeutic massage, or acupuncture. The majority of those who sought professional care from CAM providers also saw a medical doctor during the reference year. The study also observed that users of CAM therapies made almost twice as many visits to conventional medical providers as non-CAM users.

Astin (1998) conducted a mail survey of 1,035 randomly selected individuals. Forty percent of those responding (response rate 69 percent) reported CAM use during the previous year. Another survey reported by Druss and Rosenheck (1999) investigated the association between the use of CAM therapies and the use of conventional care in a different national survey sample taken from the 1996 Medical Expenditure Panel survey. They reported that in 1996 an estimated 6.5 percent of the U.S. population visited both CAM providers and conventional medical practitioners. Fewer than 2 percent used only CAM services, 60 percent used only conventional care, and 32 percent used neither. These numbers were considerably lower than the range reported by Eisenberg et al. (1998). The investigators concluded that, from the health services perspective, practitioner-based CAM therapies appear to serve more as a complement than as an alternative to conventional medical care.

In 1999, the National Health Interview Survey (NHIS) included questions about the use of alternative health care practices. Ni et al. (2002) analyzed the data from the 1999 NHIS which included 30,801 respondents and an oversampling of non-English speakers and those without telephones. A total of 12 types of CAM were asked about in the survey. Ni et al. documented a CAM use prevalence rate of 28.9 percent during the prior 12 months. The investigators concluded that on the basis of these data in 1999, CAM use was somewhat lower than that in previous surveys. Most CAM therapies were used in conjunction with conventional medical services, a finding consistent with prior observations. Lastly, the investigators pointed out that the discrepancies in overall prevalence of CAM use may largely result from the lack of agreement in the definitions of "complementary and alternative medicine."

The lack of consensus regarding a definition as to what is or what is not to be included in the category of complementary and alternative medicine has unquestionably complicated efforts to document, in a consistent fashion, the prevalence, patterns, and costs of CAM use by the American public.

Barnes and colleagues (2004) performed the most recent national analysis of CAM use using data from the 2002 NHIS. The survey included 31,044 respondents, drawn from a nationally representative sample. The 2002 survey expanded on the CAM-related questions asked in 1999, inquiring about 27 types of CAM therapies, the condition being treated, the reasons for choosing a CAM therapy, whether insurance covered the CAM therapy, the level of satisfaction with the treatment, and whether the individual's conventional medical practitioner knew about the patient's CAM use. As with previous surveys, clearly defining CAM had a large impact on the prevalence results. When "prayer for one's own health" was included in the definition, Barnes et al. found that 75 percent of adults had ever used CAM and that 62 percent of adults had used some form of CAM therapy within the past 12 months. Excluding prayer from the definition decreased the rate of CAM use to 36 percent.

The 2002 NHIS did not collect data about how much money is spent on CAM therapies, but it did report that 13 percent of CAM users chose CAM because conventional medicine was too expensive.

The patterns of CAM use described above are all based on nationally representative random samples of the adult U.S. population. As such, their results are more generalizable than data obtained from smaller clinic- and community-based surveys, which typically focus on specific health problems and specific age cohorts (Bair et al., 2002; Davis and Darden, 2003; Lee et al., 2000a), ethnic groups or geographic areas (Cushman et al., 1999; Factor-Litvak et al., 2001; Greendale et al., 2003; Maskarinec et al., 2000; Najm et al., 2003; Vallerand et al., 2003), and special at-risk populations, such as homeless youth (Breuner et al., 1998). These smaller surveys, along with qualitative studies provide insights into the health-care seeking behaviors of local populations.

USE BY POPULATION SUBGROUPS

Women

The use of CAM therapies is more common among women (48.9 percent) than men (37.8 percent) (Eisenberg et al., 1998). Wootton and Sparber (2001a,b,c) also noted this trend in their review of surveys on CAM use, as did Barnes et al. (2004) in their survey. The fact that women use CAM therapies more commonly than men is noteworthy. Women's greater use of health care services in general has been critically examined in the health social science literature in relation to such variables as social class, longevity, patterns of morbidity, symptom reporting, psychosocial distress, and gender-based differences in health care provision (Bertakis et al., 2000; Gijsbers van Wijk et al., 1992; Macintyre et al., 1996; Mustard et al., 1998). Two observations are relevant. First, women tend to be more health conscious than men leading them to invest more time and resources in promotive and preventive health (Hibbard and Pope, 1983; Verbrugge and Wingard, 1987). Second, women tend to serve as domestic health care managers influencing the health care behavior of family members, particularly when they are ill and at home (Barnett and Baruch, 1987; Carpenter, 1980; Clark, 1995; Michelson, 1990; Umberson, 1992; Verbrugge, 1989). This suggests that women's use of CAM modalities may well serve as an indicator of probable family use of CAM in the future.

Education and Income

Eisenberg and colleagues (1998) found that CAM use was higher among those who had some college education (50.6 percent) than among those with no college education (36.4 percent) and was more common among people with annual incomes above $50,000 (48.1 percent) than among those with lower incomes (42.6 percent). Foster et al. (2000), who examined a different aspect of the database of Eisenberg et al. (1998), explored the relationship between income and CAM use. They observed that complementary therapy use varied by income quartile (43 percent CAM use among those with annual incomes less than $20,000; 37 percent among those earning $20,000 to $30,000 per year; 44 percent among those earning $30,000 to $50,000 per year; and 48 percent among those with annual incomes above $50,000). In addition, the average annual out-of-pocket expenditures increased with income quartile confirming that those with higher incomes used more CAM therapies overall. Interestingly, although the data indicating that CAM use appears to be highest among those with more financial resources, the data also show that 43 percent of those in the lowest income group (those with incomes less than $20,000 per year) used CAM therapies routinely, suggesting that CAM use is prevalent in all socio-demographic segments of society (Eisenberg et al., 1998).

In the Astin (1998) survey, level of education was positively correlated with CAM use. Astin reported that 31 percent of survey participants with a high school education or less used CAM, and the rate of use increased to 50 percent for participants with a graduate degree. Household income was not a predictive factor of use, and as in the analysis of Foster et al. (2000), Astin found CAM use to be prevalent at multiple socio-demographic levels, ranging from 33 percent among those with incomes <$12,500 to 44 percent among those with incomes >$40,000.

Wootton and Sparber (2001) found that CAM users are primarily middle-aged, better educated, and in higher income brackets. However, they report that little is known about the rate of use among the less well to do since only a few small-scale studies of CAM use by low-income groups exist. Their analysis of these small-scale studies found that 29 percent (n = 199) of patients on Medicaid in a family health center used CAM; 70 percent (n = 157) of homeless young people in the Street Clinic youth program in Seattle, Washington, reported using CAM; and 56 percent (n = 187) of patients attending a family practice clinic reported using herbs/supplements.

For many types of CAM therapies, Barnes et al. (2004) found that the rate of use increased as the level of education increased. This pattern was seen for biologically based therapies, alternative medical systems, energy therapies, and manipulative and body-based therapies. The analysis of CAM use by income revealed an interaction between the type of therapy and income. Individuals who were poor[1] exhibited a slightly higher prevalence of megavitamin therapy and prayer use than individuals who were not poor (65.5 and 62.6 percent, respectively). However, individuals who were not poor reported higher rates of use of biologically based therapies (excluding megavitamin therapy), mind-body therapies (excluding prayer), alternative medical systems, energy therapies, and manipulative and body-based therapies than poor individuals.

---

[1] "Poverty" was defined by the Census Bureau's 2001 thresholds. "Poor" was defined as an income below the poverty threshold, and "not poor" was defined as an income ≥200 percent of the poverty threshold.

Ethnicity and Culture

Eisenberg and colleagues (1998) found CAM use to be less common among African Americans (33.1 percent) than among members of other racial groups (44.5 percent). In Wootton and Sparber's 2001a review, Dominican patients in an emergency room reported 50 percent use of CAM (n = 50); 94.6 percent (n = 75) of Chinese immigrants reported self-treatment and the use of home remedies; 62 percent (n = 300) of Navajos visiting an Indian Health Service hospital reported that they had used native healers; and 44 percent (n = 213) of Mexican Americans in a convenience sample reported that they had used herbal remedies, and 13 percent reported that they had used *curanderismo*.

Mackenzie and colleagues (2003) further examined the prevalence of CAM use among many different ethnic groups in the United States. They analyzed a subset of data from the 1995 National Comparative Survey of Minority Health Care of The Commonwealth Fund, a national probability sample of 3,789 people with an oversampling of ethnic minorities. The survey was conducted by telephone in six languages. The use of five categories of CAM within the last year were queried (herbal medicine, acupuncture, chiropractic, traditional healer, and home remedy). Overall, 43.1 percent of the respondents reported using one or more of those five CAM modalities. The use of CAM was equally prevalent among white, African-American/black, Latino, Asian, and Native American populations; but the characteristics of the users varied considerably by specific CAM modality. The predictors of CAM use were female gender, being uninsured, and having a high school education or above. These factors were consistent with earlier surveys involving random samples of all U.S. adults.

Ni and colleagues (2002) found that overall CAM use was higher for white non-Hispanic individuals (30.8 percent) than for Hispanic (19.9 percent) and black non-Hispanic (24.1 percent) individuals. Like the findings of Mackenzie et al. (2003), the 2002 NHIS (Barnes et al., 2004) found various patterns of use by race, depending on the type of CAM therapy. Use of mind-body therapies including prayer for health reasons was more prevalent among black adults (68.3 percent) than among white (50.1 percent) or Asian (48.1 percent) adults. However, Asian adults (43.1 percent) were more likely to use CAM (excluding megavitamin therapy and prayer) than white (35.9 percent) or black (26.2 percent) adults. Finally, white adults (12 percent) were more likely to use manipulative and body-based therapies than Asian (7.2 percent) or black (4.4 percent) adults.

It may be, however, that surveys of minority cultures underestimate health practices such as the use of home remedies since in many cultures, the consumption of foods (including commonly used herbs and spices) for medicinal purposes is so engrained in everyday folk dietetic practices that it is not recognized as being out of the ordinary or worth reporting. The same may be true for religious-spiritual practices, which serve multiple purposes and which may be reported only under extraordinary circumstances and not as routine ways of coping with adversity or ensuring well-being. There is often a fine line between what members of a minority culture deem normative practice and what outsiders classify as CAM practice. In large surveys with representative samples, there is a need for better, more culturally sensitive questions that will provide more accurate data about CAM use among minority populations.

Age

In earlier surveys, people aged 35 to 49 years reported higher rates of CAM use (50.1 percent) than people either older (39.1 percent) or younger (41.8 percent) (Eisenberg et al., 1998). Recently, the 2002 NHIS results indicate that CAM use increases with age. Barnes et al. (2004) found that 53.5 percent of the individuals in the youngest age bracket (18 to 29 years) reported that they had used some type of CAM[2] and the greatest prevalence of CAM use (70.3 percent) was found among those in the oldest age bracket (85 years and older). Wootton and Sparber's (2001a) review found that the rate of CAM use among elderly individuals ranged from 33 percent of a convenience sample of elderly patients with cancer (n = 699) to 84 percent of a convenience sample of elderly rural women. Foster et al. (2000), using the data of Eisenberg et al. (1998), measured the prevalence, cost, and patterns of CAM use by people aged 65 or older. They observed that during the previous 12 months 30 percent had used at least one type of CAM therapy for the treatment of their principal medical conditions. The complementary modalities most commonly used by individuals aged 65 and older used were chiropractic, herbal remedies and dietary supplements, relaxation and meditation techniques, and high-dose vitamins. As was the case for the general population, the majority of older adults who used CAM services made no mention of this to their physician.

Fewer studies have examined the use of CAM by children. Davis and Darden (2003) analyzed a 1996 nationally representative survey of American children and reported a prevalence rate of 1.8 percent. Among CAM users, 76.8 percent were white and 54 percent were female. CAM use increased with age, with older children (ages 10 to 17 years) accounting for 62.6 percent of the use, but the youngest children (ages 0 to 4 years) representing only 21 percent. The investigators noted that the overall estimate of CAM use was lower than that reported in previous surveys and

---

[2]CAM use included megavitamin therapy and prayer.

discussed possible explanations. Like other national surveys, CAM is not defined consistently among surveys. This particular survey asked whether a CAM provider was consulted in the previous year, which does not take into account the use of self-prescribed therapies, such as dietary supplements.

TYPES OF ILLNESS

Studies of the use of CAM for the treatment of specific illnesses have documented the popularity of CAM for the treatment of health problems that lack definitive cures; that have an unpredictable course and prognosis; and that are associated with substantial pain, discomfort, or side effects from prescription drug medicine. For example, back pain/back problem was the most common condition (16.8 percent) identified in the 2002 NHIS (Barnes et al., 2004). CAM use has been identified as particularly common among women suffering from the symptoms of menopause (Beal, 1998; Cherrington et al., 2003; Kronenberg and Fugh-Berman, 2002) and pregnancy-related illnesses (Tiran, 2002), gynecology problems (von Gruenigen et al., 2001), rheumatology problems (Rao et al., 1999; Wootton and Sparber, 2001c), gastroenterological diseases (Rawsthorne et al., 1999), rhinosinusitis (Krouse and Krouse, 1999), attention and hyperactivity problems (Chan et al., 2003), psychiatric and neurological problems (Sparber and Wootton, 2002), cancer (Adler, 1999; Bernstein and Grasso, 2001; Burstein et al., 1999; Henderson and Donatelle, 2004; Kao and Devine, 2000; Lee et al., 2002; Lee et al., 2000b; Lengacher et al., 2002; Patterson et al., 2002; Richardson et al., 2000, Sparber and Wootton, 2001; Sparber et al., 2000; Swisher et al., 2002; VandeCreek et al., 1999; Wilkinson et al., 2002; Zimmerman and Thompson, 2002), HIV/AIDS (Fairfield et al., 1998; Wootton and Sparber, 2001b), asthma (Braganza et al., 2003), and disabilities (Krauss et al., 1998). Still other studies have examined the prevalence of patients who use CAM in various types of nonspecialty clinics such as pediatric clinics (Davis and Darden, 2003; Madsen et al., 2003; Sawni-Sikand et al., 2002), primary-care clinics (Gordon et al., 1998; Kitai et al., 1998), maternity practices (Hepner et al., 2002), emergency rooms (Gulla and Singer, 2000; Rogers et al., 2001; Weiss et al., 2001), and postsurgery clinics (Norred et al., 2000). One reason for conducting such studies has been to identify possible CAM-conventional medicine interactions, especially in cases in which it is vital to a patient's well-being to know of medications that may interfere with such things as blood clotting time when surgery is being performed (Allaire et al., 2000; Hepner et al., 2002) or with other conventional practices that have been taken or have been prescribed by CAM practitioners or midwives.

These examples are not meant to be exhaustive but, rather, representative of the range of studies that have used various sampling techniques and that have been performed with particular U.S. patient populations over the past decade. These surveys confirm the impression that a significant percentage of individuals with chronic or life-threatening illnesses are using CAM at some point during the course of their illness.

More difficult to discern are an individual's reasons for using a CAM modality at a particular point in time over the course of an illness. One cannot tell from survey data whether those surveyed used a CAM modality primarily for curative purposes or primarily for a specific health problem, as a means of reducing the side effects from other types of therapy, or for general health-promoting purposes. Nor can it be determined which type of therapy (conventional or CAM) was sought first. It is worth noting that for many of the chronic conditions listed above, management of patients' health care needs includes but extends beyond the management of overt symptoms associated with the disease. The importance of this observation may be considered in light of studies on health care expenditures associated with chronic disease. It has been estimated that more than 45 percent of noninstitutionalized Americans have one or more chronic conditions and their direct health care costs account for 75 percent of U.S. health care expenditures (Hoffman et al., 1996).

Using a nationally representative sample of 23,230 U.S. residents, Druss et al. (2001) calculated that half of U.S. health care costs in 1996 were borne by persons with one or more of five conditions: mood disorders, diabetes, heart disease, asthma, and hypertension. Notably, of that amount, only about one-quarter was spent on treating the conditions themselves; the remainder was spent on treating coexistent illnesses and health care problems. Those researchers pointed out that each condition was associated with unique patterns of health service use driving those costs. This finding highlights the need for a better understanding of what motivates patients with chronic complaints to seek both CAM and conventional medical services and the cost implications of combined care. In other words, does utilization of CAM reduce or increase the costs of health care for people with different types of chronic conditions?

FREQUENCY OF USE

Wolsko and colleagues (2002), using the database of Eisenberg et al. (1998), evaluated the extent to which high-frequency users of CAM contributed to the total number of visits to CAM providers. Notably, they found that individuals who saw conventional health care providers more frequently were also the most apt to use complementary care services. Conservative extrapolation to national estimates suggested that a small fraction of U.S. adults (8.9 percent) accounted for 20 percent of CAM users but that they made more than 75 percent of the 629 million visits to CAM providers. These data parallel observations that a large percentage of the annual U.S. health care budget is routinely consumed by a relatively small percentage of the U.S. population. CAM services can and should be viewed similarly. Notably, however, high-frequency users of biomedicine and high-frequency users of CAM appear to use these modalities for different purposes. Additionally, Druss and Rosenheck (1999) point to a difference between these two populations of high-frequency users: psychiatric disorders are prominent among the high-frequency users of conventional medicine, but the researchers found no such correlate among high-frequency users of CAM modalities.

Wolsko and colleagues (2002) also examined the extent to which insurance coverage was independently associated with CAM therapy use. They found that for individuals who sought the services of practitioners who performed physical manipulation (e.g., chiropractors and massage therapists), full insurance coverage, partial insurance coverage, and the use of the therapy for wellness were all associated with the high-frequency use of such providers. Among the survey respondents using the services of CAM providers, 63 percent of those reporting that they had full insurance coverage made eight or more visits to a CAM practitioner during the previous year. Only 17 percent of those reporting that they had no insurance coverage made eight or more visits. For CAM therapies which were not related to physical manipulation (e.g., relaxation therapy and advice regarding herbs supplements), the only factor associated with high-frequency provider use was having used the therapy for wellness. Having any insurance coverage, it appears, is associated with higher rates of use of CAM therapy services. Rates of insurance coverage for CAM services varies significantly by state, treatment plan, and CAM modality (Tillman, 2002). The services of chiropractors are covered by between 41 and 65 percent of health maintenance organizations (HMOs), the services of homeopaths are covered by 4 to 11 percent of HMOs, acupuncture is covered by 9 to 19 percent of HMOs, and massage therapy is covered by 6 to 10 percent of HMOs (Stanger and Coughlan, 2000). Depending on the therapy, Eisenberg et al. (1998) also found various rates of partial and full coverage, with only four modalities (chiropractic, megavitamins, imagery, and biofeedback) receiving some form of coverage more than 50 percent of the time.

LONG-TERM TRENDS IN CAM USE

What are the long-term trends in CAM use likely to be and how do they differ from the trends experienced earlier in history? Kessler and colleagues (2001) analyzed the same dataset obtained by Eisenberg et al. (1998) in their 1997 survey, but focused on questions about first-time use of CAM therapies by all individuals aged 18 and older. They observed that 68 percent of all respondents had used as least one CAM therapy during the course of their lives. Lifetime use steadily increased with age across all age cohorts. Specifically, individuals in the pre-baby boom cohort (i.e., older than age 58 years at the time of the survey) had a 30 percent incidence of CAM therapy use by the age of 33; 5 of 10 baby boomers had used one or more CAM therapies by age 33, and 7 of 10 individuals born after the baby boom reported the use of some type of CAM therapy by age 33. It was also noted that prior use of any CAM therapy was an excellent predictor of current use. Among the respondents who had ever used a CAM therapy, roughly half continued to use a CAM therapy many years later (during the interval of the survey).

These analyses also documented the fact that the rate of use of all but 4 of the 20 most commonly used complementary therapies increased in frequency beginning in the 1960s. During the decades of the 1970s, 1980s, and 1990s, the use of particular CAM therapies increased at higher rates than the use of others. For instance, the 1970s witnessed large increases in the rates of use of herbal medicine, imagery, energy healing and biofeedback, whereas in the 1980s the rates of use of massage therapy and naturopathy increased most rapidly.

Kessler and colleagues (2001) mention that "from an historical perspective, data from 1998 may not necessarily represent a consistent trend of increased use of CAM therapies, but rather a distinct peak in a long trend of constant fluctuation in complementary and alternative medicine use by the American public." They refer to previous peaks of CAM use such as survey data from the 1920s and 1930s indicating high rates of use of "unconventional" therapies and government statistics from 1900 documenting large numbers of registered "alternative" practitioners. Kessler et al. conclude that the recent high rates of CAM use may in fact be demonstrating a resurgence of CAM use after a period of diminished use during the 1940s and 50s. Even so, use of CAM therapies in recent years by a large proportion of the U.S. population is seen as a result of a historical trend that began at least 50 years ago. Moreover, this trend suggests a continuing demand for CAM therapies that will affect health care delivery for the foreseeable future.

Other factors associated with CAM therapy use that further this hypothesis include the observation that CAM therapies are used predominantly for the treatment of chronic disease, which, as mentioned above, accounts for an increasing fraction of the U.S. healthcare burden (Astin, 1998). In addition, an estimated one-third of CAM therapy use is attributed to disease prevention and health promotion (Eisenberg et al., 1993, 1998). These patterns parallel trends in U.S. society to promote disease prevention and to encourage health promotion, especially among those in the baby boom generation, 50 percent of whom already use CAM therapies, usually in the absence of a chronic or a disabling disease. As such, CAM use is quite likely to increase in the coming quarter century as the baby boom generation experiences greater disease burdens. Lastly, the observation that 7 of 10 individuals born after the baby boom generation routinely use CAM therapies by the age of 33 (Kessler et al., 2001) suggests that the U.S. public increasingly views CAM therapies as accessible options and "conventional" lifestyle choices that can no longer be viewed as entirely "alternative" practices.

COST-EFFECTIVENESS

CAM therapies are typically not centered on high-technology interventions and instead include low-cost treatments. This is often offered in support of the idea that CAM may provide more cost-effective treatments than conventional medicine. However, some CAM interventions involve more time with a practitioner, which may be costly (White and Ernst, 2000). Despite the claim that CAM is more cost-effective, there is not a large body of literature that explores the question of cost. White and Ernst (2000) conducted a review of cost description, cost comparison, cost-effectiveness, and cost-benefit studies. The studies in the articles reviewed tended to take two general approaches: evaluation of the cost of a specific therapy and health condition and examination of overall effects, such as rates and total health care costs. With a few exceptions, White and Ernst did not find a rigorous body of economic analyses for CAM. They offer several explanations, including the "intangible and indirect" benefits of CAM, such as patient preference, patient empowerment, and quality of life, as well as the cumulative benefits conveyed through lifestyle changes.

Since the review of White and Ernst (2000) was published, a few more economic evaluations of CAM have been published. Sobel (2000) reviewed four examples of mind-body interventions that demonstrated beneficial effects on health and cost-savings for heart disease, chronic disease, surgery, and prematurity among infants. For chronic low back pain, Cherkin et al. (2001) compared the effectiveness of acupuncture, massage, and self-care education. At the 1-year follow-up, patients randomized to receive therapeutic massage reported fewer symptoms than acupuncture recipients, and massage recipients used fewer medications than the other two groups. Finally, follow-up costs for outpatient HMO back care were lower for the massage group than for the acupuncture or the education group, although the difference was not statistically significant. An important limitation of this study was the lack of a no-treatment comparison group.

The treatment of chronic headaches with acupuncture was the subject of a recent randomized clinical trial and cost-effectiveness analysis by Wonderling and colleagues (2004) in the United Kingdom. Compared with usual care, acupuncture increased both quality-adjusted life years[3] and health care costs. However, the investigators noted that the cost increase is less than that of another National Health Service-recommended medication for the treatment of migraine headaches. A second randomized controlled trial paired with an economic analysis, conducted in The Netherlands, examined the treatment of neck pain with physiotherapy, manual therapy, and general practitioner care (Korthals-de Bos et al., 2003). At 26 weeks, manual therapy led to a faster recovery. Additionally, at the 1-year follow-up, the analysis showed that manual therapy (i.e., spinal mobilization) cost less and was more effective than physiotherapy (i.e., mainly exercise) or general care (i.e., counseling, education, and medication). It should be emphasized that few studies of the cost-effectiveness of CAM therapies have been undertaken.

WHAT MOTIVATES PEOPLE TO USE CAM

Survey techniques are useful for finding out the personal and demographic characteristics of people who have tried CAM modalities, the point prevalence rate of people who have used CAM over specified periods of time (ever, last year, etc.), how much they have spent on these modalities, where they have received therapy (if they saw a CAM practitioner) or if they have engaged in self-treatment, and whether they have informed their conventional medical doctor that they are using CAM therapies or modalities (or whether they have informed their CAM practitioner that they are receiving biomedical treatments). They are far less useful as a means of providing information about people's motivations for using CAM therapies or modalities, given that rationale and rationalization are hard to tease apart on a survey and given that the reasons for using CAM use change over time, are complex, and are multidimensional.

A wide variety of motivations for using CAM have been reported in the literature dispelling any simple characterization of why the American public uses CAM therapies and modalities. Table 2-2 identifies many of the motivations for the use of CAM that have been identified in the health, social science, and CAM literature (Astin, 1998; Easthope, 1986; Foote-Ardah, 2003; Furnham and Forey, 1994; Furnham and Smith, 1988; Henderson and Donatelle, 2004; Kaptchuck and Eisenberg, 1998; Kelner and Wellman, 1997; Lloyd et al., 1993; Mitchell and Cormack, 1998;

---

[3]"Quality-adjusted life years integrate mortality and morbidity to express health status in terms of equivalents of well-years of life" (Kaplan, 1988).

Sharma, 1992, 1996; Siahpush, 1999; Sirois and Glick, 2002; Sollner et al., 2000; Thorne et al., 2002).

An important finding noted by Wolsko et al. (2002) was that among the 2,055 study participants, the pursuit of wellness was a major contributor to CAM use. Those who used CAM for wellness purposes frequented CAM providers more often than those who did not. Other researchers have also noted that interest in health promotion and disease prevention appears to be a motivating force driving CAM use (Astin, 1998). Research suggests that obtaining "wellness care" from conventional and CAM providers is important to CAM users. Druss and Rosenheck (1999) found that adults who visit both CAM providers and conventional providers are more likely than individuals who seek care only from conventional providers to report that they monitor their blood pressure and cholesterol levels and undertake timely prostate and breast cancer screenings.

Astin and colleagues (2000) surveyed enrollees in a Medicare supplement plan offering benefits for selected CAM therapies and found that the most frequently cited reason for CAM use was "general health improvement" (42 percent), whereas CAM use for "chronic medical problems" was cited by only 18 percent of those surveyed. These findings are consistent with the findings of Eisenberg et al. (1993, 1998), who documented that 58 percent of those surveyed used CAM therapies, at least in part, to "prevent future illness from occurring or to maintain health and vitality," whereas only 42 percent of those surveyed used CAM exclusively to treat an existing disease.

The 2002 NHIS asked participants about their reasons for using CAM. For any type of CAM, 54.9 percent believed that CAM therapy combined with conventional medical treatments would help, 50.1 percent thought that CAM would be interesting to try and 25.8 percent indicated that CAM use was suggested by a conventional medical professional. Alternatively, 27.7 percent believed that conventional medical treatments would not help, and 13.2 percent believed that conventional medical therapies were too expensive (Barnes et al., 2004).

Once a patient begins to use CAM therapies, however, how likely is the patient to continue to use them? Cross-sectional surveys carried out after time lapses of some years allow investigators to speculate about continued use for some purpose, be it health promotion, the treatment of periodic illness, or the management of a chronic illness or disability. Kessler et al. (2001) found that 50 percent of all CAM therapy use that had been initiated at least 5 years prior to the interview (Eisenberg et al., 1998) persisted at the time of the interview. This suggests that prior use of CAM therapy is a predictor of ongoing or current use for half of all users. The data also suggest that the persistent use of CAM therapies and modalities may be related to general health and may not be reserved only for the treatment of

TABLE 2-2 Reasons Why Different Types of People Use CAM Modalities at Different Points in Their Lives

User	Reasons for Using CAM or User Characteristic
Experimenter open to new experience	Try and see, nothing to lose, may just help attitude
Those heavily influenced by the commodification of health	Responds to the health claims of CAM no differently from the response to other health products; to stay healthy one consumes health products
Heavy users of all systems of medicine and types of practitioners	Is either very health conscious or derives secondary gain from seeking help, or may use care-seeking as an idiom of distress or as a way of mobilizing support
Enlightened users of CAM	Embraces the principles underlying the ethnomedicine or subscribes to these principles to the point that they influence lifestyle as well as the treatment of particular illnesses; the ideology of the CAM system may be embraced as a form of spiritual (or spiritual materialist) practice or as a philosophy
Seekers of new cure for an old problem that persists	Conventional medicine does not work well for the complaint
Those afflicted with a chronic illness, disease or disability	CAM enables the patient to play a more active and participatory role in care, assume greater responsibility, and obtain an increasing sense of control; provides a new diagnostic label more in keeping with the patient's view of the illness; a new label may gain legitimization for a complaint not diagnosed by biomedicine; use driven by sense that one has been misdiagnosed or underdiagnosed by conventional medicine; the patient is looking for other ways to understand illness to make the experience more coherent; a shift in meaning entails a shift in the sense of responsibility
	CAM enables the patient to manage and reserve valued conventional medications (e.g., antiretroviral medications) until they are really needed—extending the duration of their effectiveness; reduction of side effects from conventional medicine (for patients with

TABLE 2-2 Continued

User	Reasons for Using CAM or User Characteristic
	acute and chronic illnesses); to prevent disease recurrence and improve quality of life
Those who mistrust the health care system as looking out for their best interests at a time of cost cutting and austerity	Lack of trust in and disenchantment with health care system which has not met expectations
Those who maintain a cynical view that biomedicine can treat or manage a particular condition	Dissatisfaction with previous treatment outcomes based on previous experiences
Those dissatisfied by doctor-patient relationship because of the interaction, a lack of communication, and or limited time	Looking for more patient-centered approach to the treatment of illness which fits the treatment to the patient's life and what is valued by the patient; a more caring and closer practitioner-patient relationship that affords personal attention is sought
Those interested in promoting wellness	Use of CAM to enhance energy, reestablish a sense of balance or rhythm, increase resistance, increase immunity, and reduce stress
"Harm reduction" user	Reduces harm of unhealthy workplace, environment, lifestyle, etc.
"Needs an edge" user	Expressed in terms of energy, focus, memory, and enhanced abilities
"Can't afford to be ill" user	CAM is a promotive or preventive health aid to ward off illness especially when feeling vulnerable
Those who have limited access to conventional medicine and who cannot afford it except for cases of severe illness	CAM serves as a stop-gap function and is used as just another form of over-the-counter medicine
Those who are able to mobilize social support	By being involved with CAM one enlarges, solidifies or mobilizes his or her support network
Those encouraged by friends or family to try CAM	Direct and indirect influence by people who have heard that the CAM modality can help
Those able to take personal time through CAM use	Self-care is justified; one is able to focus on self and secure personal time
Those making a lifestyle statement	CAM use is part of bigger package and identity; the person may or may not understand the ethnomedical system, but does approve of what it stands for: meaning is derived from participation with the modality

continued

TABLE 2-2 Continued

User	Reasons for Using CAM or User Characteristic
Those who are fighting aging, trying to stay young user	CAM use is related to wide range of functions from retaining or enhancing beauty or flexibility to increasing vitality or removing toxins associated with the aging process
Those skeptical of CAM	The user does not have positive expectations, but is trying anyway; some users maintain negative expectations that they await to be disproved
Those unaware they are using CAM	Many consumers of dietary supplements are unaware that what they are taking is not medicine recommended or approved by conventional medicine

a particular time-limited ailment. This is consistent with the findings of Astin (1998) that most CAM therapies are used, at least in part, to prevent future illness or to maintain health and vitality as part of lifestyle choices linked to disease prevention and health promotion.

Further investigation into the association between the use of CAM modalities and wellness-related behavior is warranted given national public health priorities and the burden of lifestyle-related diseases (DHHS, 2000). What remains unknown is the extent to which different types and levels of CAM use foster or sustain behavioral changes contributing to positive health outcomes. CAM use may be a marker of "packages" of lifestyle changes associated with shifts in identity, or it may constitute little more than an attempt at harm reduction engaged by those who wish to minimize the negative effects of an unhealthy environment, job, or lifestyle (Nichter, 2003). Data on wellness from existing cross-sectional surveys point out the need for long-term longitudinal cohort studies examining large numbers of adults who are routinely asked questions about CAM use as well as diet, exercise, smoking, etc. Such studies, reminiscent of the Framingham Heart Study or the Nurses' Health Study (both of which are ongoing and which could, conceivably, be expanded to include questions about CAM use) may offer the best opportunity to explore patterns of CAM use over time as well as the role—or lack thereof—of CAM in promoting health, reducing risk, and preventing disease.

One hypothesis for why people use CAM is that they are dissatisfied with conventional care. The literature suggests that this is not most user's primary reason for CAM use (Astin, 1998; Barnes et al., 2004; Eisenberg et al., 2001). Users of CAM often use CAM modalities simultaneously with conventional medicine when they are ill. They typically (70 percent) use CAM subsequent to or simultaneously with the use of conventional medicine, and 79 percent of respondents who saw a medical doctor and used CAM therapies perceived the combination to be superior to either one alone (Eisenberg et al., 2001). A second hypothesis is that CAM users maintain health beliefs different from those of other people, but an answer to this question will require investigation of health perceptions before and after CAM use to determine whether users sought CAM modalities on the basis of their health ideology or underwent transformational experiences.

Astin (1998) conducted the only national survey on personal factors that predispose individuals to use CAM. He found that higher levels of education, a transformational experience that changed one's world view, a holistic health philosophy, and interest in alternative lifestyles were determinants of CAM use. Other studies have also documented an association between CAM use and a holistic (e.g., New Age) health philosophy (Easthope et al., 2000; Furnham and Forey, 1994; Pawluch et al., 2000; Sharma, 1993). Although embracing such a philosophy is undoubtedly a factor related to sustained CAM use by many people, it is most likely not the initial motivation for many others to seek care from CAM practitioners or to use CAM-related resources (Kelner and Wellman, 1997).

The research summarized in Table 2-2 suggests that people seek CAM modalities for a wide variety of reasons. Some of those attracted to CAM modalities seek a therapeutic relationship with a practitioner in which they have the opportunity to more fully participate in their own health care decision making (Mitchell and Cormack, 1998). For example, cancer patients vary considerably in their preference for participation in decision making. While some of those who wish to share responsibility for care find preferred relationships with practitioners of conventional medicine, many others do not (Arora, 2003). Many who use CAM as supplementary care do so as a way of avoiding passivity and coping with feelings of hopelessness. It might be more productive to investigate the extent to which these individuals are simply trying to marshal all resources at their disposal toward the end of securing optimal health care, a concept that is relative and subject to interpretation in accord with a patient's needs and expectations.

For many people, all forms of health care are options, alternatives to be exploited in an everexpanding health care arena subject to market forces, scientific evolution, and the vagaries of public opinion. Many CAM users access different forms of health care from different places with limited if any coordination between practitioners or knowledge being shared about the eclectic therapies used or medicines taken. Lack of coordination is far from ideal. Research needs to address the multiple factors motivating health care seeking in the pluralistic health care arena that exists at present and the use of eclectic health care resources by the American public.

One problem with general characterizations of why people use CAM is that such representations overlook different motivations for initiating CAM and sustaining CAM use over time. They also generate stereotypes about CAM and conventional practitioners that are simplistic and not borne out by the evidence. Figure 2-1 summarizes information from a nationally representative sample on how dual users of CAM and conventional medicine compare these two broad types of health care and their interactions with both types of care providers. Figure 2-1 depicts a very mixed picture of how users of CAM feel about their practitioners (Eisenberg et al., 1998).

Motivations for using CAM change over time and are influenced by many potentially important intervening variables: frustrations with existing therapies, a desire to try something new, changes in the meaning that one attributes to one's ailment, changes in self-identity associated with CAM use, the economics of receiving care, and the feedback that one receives from significant others who form an individual's therapy management support group. The user types highlighted in Table 2-2 represent a heuristic. Real users of CAM are likely to approximate different ideal types at different points in their lives as well as to be influenced by multiple motivations to use CAM at any one time.

Sirois and Gick (2002) have recently called for a more sophisticated way of looking at CAM users that does not treat them as a homogeneous group with similar beliefs, motivations, and needs and that attends to how their behaviors change over time. They conducted one of the few studies to explore differences in the reasons for using CAM among two groups of CAM users, defined by the length and frequency of CAM use, and a comparison group of users of conventional medicine. New or infrequent CAM users, established CAM users, and users of conventional medicine were distinguished on the basis of health beliefs and sociodemographic, medical, and personality variables. Different patterns of predictors of CAM use for the different groups emerged. In general, health-aware behaviors and dissatisfaction with conventional medicine were the best predictors of overall and initial or infrequent CAM use, while more frequent health-aware behaviors were associated with continued CAM use. Medical need also influenced the choice to use CAM and was the best predictor of committed CAM use, with the established CAM users reporting more health problems than the group of new or infrequent CAM users. An openness to new experiences was associated with CAM use, most notably in the decision to initially try or explore the use of CAM. In a further analysis of their data, Sirois (2002) found that newer CAM users still relied heavily on conventional medical treatments, whereas more experienced CAM users depended

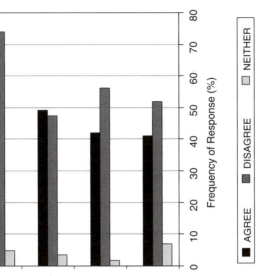

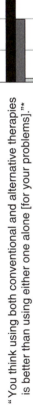

FIGURE 2.1 Users' comparison of CAM and conventional health care.

NOTE: * Asked of respondents who had seen a medical doctor and used any CAM therapies (including use of self prayer alone) in the past 12 months.†Asked of respondents who had seen both CAM therapy providers and medical doctors within the past 12 months.
SOURCE: Eisenberg et al., 2001.

less on CAM alone and more on CAM for the treatment of their non-life-threatening health problems.

ACCESSING INFORMATION ABOUT CAM

Little research has been carried out to investigate

- Where the public goes to search for information about CAM modalities
- What sources of information they commonly find and access
- The effect of CAM advertising on health care seeking behavior
- What types of the information are deemed credible, marginal, and spurious
- How risks and benefits are understood and how such perceptions inform decision making
- What the public expects their providers to tell them

Information about CAM modalities appears to be obtained in three major ways. First, it has widely been reported that information about CAM is often spread by word of mouth within social networks and that referral by lay individuals is common. However, the committee found no study that investigated the impact of one person's CAM involvement on that person's immediate family or larger social network. Analysis of CAM use among those afflicted with particular health problems and those engaging in promotive health activities associated with CAM is needed.

The second source of information is the Internet. It is known that a significant percentage of the American public conducts Internet-based searches to find information about health problems and potential treatments. A recent study estimated that 73 million Americans, or 62 percent of Americans with access to the Internet at the time, have used the Internet to search for information related to health care (Fox and Rainie, 2002). Of these health information seekers, 92 percent reported that the information that they obtained during their last Internet search was useful and relevant (Fox et al., 2000), and 68 percent indicated that it had some role in their health care decision making (Fox and Rainie, 2002). It is reasonable to assume that many of those contemplating or already using CAM modalities access the Internet to find out about these modalities.

A few studies have been conducted to determine what a hypothetical health seeker might find on the Internet were he or she to search for common herbal medications. Morris and Avorn (2003) searched the Internet using the five most commonly used search engines and examined what surfaced when they entered the names of the eight most widely used herbal supplements (*Ginkgo biloba*, St. John's wort, echinacea, ginseng, garlic, saw palmetto, kava kava, and valerian root). The health content of all websites listed on the first page of the search results were analyzed for a total of 443 sites that met study inclusion criteria. Among the 443 websites, 338 (76 percent) were retail sites. Eighty-one percent of these retail websites made one or more health claims; of these, 149 (55 percent) claimed to treat, prevent, diagnose, or cure specific diseases. More than one-half (153 of 292; 52 percent) of the sites with a health claim omitted the standard federal disclaimer. Bonakdar (2002) conducted a disease-specific search for herbal drugs for cancer. A majority of sites examined claimed that they offered cures for cancer through herbal supplementation with little regard for federal regulations against doing so, with such claims being more common on sites operated from outside the United States.

Ashar and colleagues (2003) conducted a third study that evaluated information contained within Internet sites that advertise and market dietary supplements containing ephedra. Thirty-two products and advertisements were identified and systematically evaluated for deviance from truth-in-advertising standards. Of the 32 websites analyzed, 13 (41 percent) failed to disclose potential adverse effects or contraindications to supplement use. Seventeen (53 percent) did not reveal the recommended dosage of ephedra alkaloids. More importantly, 11 sites (34 percent) contained incorrect or misleading statements, some of which could directly result in serious harm to consumers. These and other studies (Matthews et al., 2003; Sagaram et al., 2002) illustrate that consumers are commonly misled by vendors' claims that herbal products can treat, prevent, diagnose, or cure specific diseases, despite regulations prohibiting such statements. Closer monitoring of web sites, enforcement of the Dietary Supplement Health and Education Act of 1994 (DSHEA) and Federal Trade Commission regulations, and the creation of a user-friendly authoritative website or criteria for evaluating existing websites on CAM modalities are much needed.

A third common source of information about CAM-related modalities is health food stores. A handful of surrogate patient studies have been conducted in which a researcher poses as a prospective client and asks for advice about what type of herbal medicine he or she (or a family member) should take for a specified ailment. In one study conducted by Mills et al. (2003), eight data gatherers asked employees of all retail health food stores in a major Canadian city what they recommended for a patient with breast cancer. The data gatherers inquired about product safety, potential drug interactions, cost, and efficacy. Employees at 34 stores were queried, and a total of 33 different products were recommended. Twenty-three employees (68 percent) did not ask whether the patient took prescription medications, 15 employees (44 percent) recommended visiting some type of health care professional, and only 3 employees (8.8 percent) discussed the potential adverse effects of the products.

In another study, Glisson et al. (2003) investigated what products health food store employees recommended for the treatment of depression and how they explained the benefits and risks. Twelve health food stores in the United States were selected for the study. An investigator approached an employee in each store and asked what he or she recommended for depression plus five additional questions regarding product use. All 12 health food store employees recommended a St. John's wort supplement for the treatment of depression. The employees made numerous comments about St. John's wort and its use for treatment of depression that were unsafe and inaccurate. Notably, that study and another study of shopkeeper recommendations for medications for children with Crohn's disease (Calder et al., 2000) found that health food store employees tend to refer to a common resource when making recommendations. If this is a widespread practice, the availability of public access to a website recognized by health food store employees as authoritative might enhance the therapeutic advice given and minimize the potential for dangerous errors to be made when they offer information, especially if the customer was asked to indicate other medications taken at the time.

HOW THE AMERICAN PUBLIC USES CAM MODALITIES

Although reliable data exist on the percentage of people who have used a CAM modality in the last year and how many times the modality was used in general, far less is known about the reasons for CAM use at various times. Existing surveys also provide little information about what proportions of CAM use are

- Self-initiated: "I go to a provider and ask for X."
- Provider initiated: "I go to a provider and she recommends or administers X."
- Provider administered: "She does X [massage, acupuncture, chiropractic] to me."
- Self-administered: "I read how to do it or someone shows me and then I do it myself in a fashion I find comfortable; I self-regulate X [herbs, self hypnosis, yoga, etc.]."

Little is known about how individual patients actually use CAM modalities while they are under the care of a CAM practitioner or engaging in self-treatment. The committee was not able to find a single scientific study to date on the rates of compliance or adherence to CAM therapies or supplements purchased over the counter. This stands in stark contrast to a rather robust literature on adherence in conventional medicine (DiMatteo et al., 2002; Donovan and Blake, 1992; Vermeire et al., 2001), a search for which on the PubMed website conducted in December 2003 yielded more than 50,000 citations.

Further, we have no information about whether or the extent to which use of a CAM therapy may interfere with compliance in the use of conventional therapies. Having no information about the extent to which patients using CAM adhere to guidelines or directions for treatment produces a major gap in our knowledge. We do not know if patients are using products as directed or even for the purpose recommended. Such information is important, not because we want to assure that patients "follow orders," but rather to assure that patients are using products and therapies safely and effectively. Even if a therapy is efficacious, it may have little or no effect if it is taken or used incorrectly. Indeed, medicines and other CAM products and procedures may be the source of iatrogenic health problems if they are used incorrectly. It has been routinely observed that a significant proportion of those who take conventional medicine are noncomplaint for a host of reasons. Nonadherence to treatment guidelines may be just as common in the case of CAM. Indeed, patients who believe that herbal medicines are harmless may be more willing to self-regulate their medication in unsupervised ways.

Studies of adherence to dietary supplements pose a special challenge. Because of government regulations (DSHEA), supplement labels are not allowed to make claims about the treatment for named illnesses, although they are commonly used for this purpose. Instructions on packages are therefore written to address complaints according to "structure and function" guidelines (see Chapter 9). At issue is whether users are following the printed instructions or are using these "medicines" for other purposes. On the other hand, are they seeking information on how to use supplements from other sources? On the basis of what criteria can compliance be ascertained? A lack of data on compliance is a major oversight in current CAM research.

Use of CAM in Supervised, Unsupervised, and Eclectic Ways

Unlike many conventional approaches to health care (e.g., prescription medications, surgical procedures, chemotherapy, and radiation), some CAM therapies are provided by licensed practitioners (e.g., acupuncturists, chiropractors, and massage therapists); others are provided by practitioners or are used by individuals without professional supervision (e.g., meditation and relaxation techniques, dietary supplementation, and dietary modification) and some forms are used without professional supervision altogether. As reported by Eisenberg et al. (1993), in 1990 nearly half (47 percent) of respondents who used one or more CAM therapies for their principal medical conditions did so without any professional supervision, that is, without either visiting a CAM practitioner or discussing their CAM therapy with their medical doctor.

It is also known that individuals who use CAM therapies tend to do so rather eclectically and in complex ways. Wolsko et al. (2002) reported that among individuals who used one or more CAM therapies in 1998, 46 percent used one therapy, 20 percent used two therapies, 13 percent used three therapies, 7 percent used four therapies, 5 percent used five therapies, 3 percent used six therapies, and 5.5 percent used seven or more therapies. Of the respondents who used CAM therapies during the prior 12 months, an estimated 48 percent used only self-care-centered CAM modalities, whereas 52 percent had seen a CAM provider. Among those who sought services of a professional CAM provider, 33 percent saw one type of CAM provider, 11 percent saw two types of CAM providers, and 8 percent saw three or more different types of CAM providers.

These findings have implications for the design of future clinical trials to assess the safety, efficacy, and cost-effectiveness of CAM therapy use by the adult population. Although it is still important to evaluate individual therapies for individual conditions, a research portfolio that is limited to this approach may not adequately simulate CAM therapy use by the adult population. It may therefore be important methodologically to design some studies that offer patients access to multiple CAM therapies across multiple CAM professional groups, as this would be closer to real-life experience.

It is also interesting to reflect on the sequence, in which adults use CAM therapies in the context of their overall health care management. Eisenberg et al. (1993, 1998) documented that the overwhelming majority of CAM users also sought conventional medical care for their principal medical conditions. In a separate analysis, Eisenberg et al. (2001) explored the sequence in which individuals seek CAM therapy and found that 70 percent of respondents typically sought the services of a CAM professional concurrently with or after their visit to a medical doctor. Less than 15 percent reported that they had seen a CAM therapy provider before an evaluation of their medical concern by a medical doctor. As such, future research may need to incorporate options for concurrent and concomitant conventional and CAM therapies for individuals to see whether one is better than the other or, alternatively, whether the two together (as usually occurs in common practice) provide perceived or real improvements in clinical outcomes or cost-effectiveness, or both.

Knowledge of the basis for decision making by the U.S. public regarding when and how they access complementary therapies either through professional contact with licensed practitioners or some form of self-care is lacking. This represents a relatively unchartered line of inquiry that also has implications for future studies in this field.

CHARACTERISTICS OF CAM THERAPIES PROVIDED BY LICENSED ACUPUNCTURISTS, CHIROPRACTORS, MASSAGE THERAPISTS, AND NATUROPATHS

Although much of the information regarding the prevalence and the patterns of CAM use comes from surveys of patients, studies of CAM practitioners aimed at documenting the types of patients whom they see and the types of therapeutic options that they offer have also been conducted. Cherkin et al. (2002a,b) surveyed random samples of licensed acupuncturists, chiropractors, massage therapists, and naturopathic physicians and collected data on the patients who visited those providers. Specifically, they collected data on 20 consecutive visits to a random sample of licensed CAM therapists in four states (Arizona, Connecticut, Massachusetts, and Washington) and compared the data with data on conventional physician visits from the National Ambulatory Medical Care Survey. The data reported came from at least 99 practitioners in each professional group and were collected for more than 1,800 ambulatory visits. More than 80 percent of the visits to CAM providers were by young and middle-aged adults, and roughly two-thirds were by women. Children made 10 percent of the visits to naturopathic physicians but only 1 to 4 percent of all visits to all other CAM providers. At least two-thirds of the visits resulted from self-referrals, and only 4 to 12 percent of the visits were a result of referrals by conventional physicians. Chiropractors and massage therapists primarily saw patients with musculoskeletal problems (e.g., patients with back, neck, and shoulder symptoms), whereas acupuncturists and naturopathic physicians saw a broader range of conditions (including fatigue, mental health issues, and headaches). Visits to acupuncturists and massage therapists lasted about 60 minutes, whereas visits to naturopathic physicians lasted 40 minutes, those to chiropractors lasted less than 20 minutes, and a routine visit with a conventional physician lasted less than 10 minutes. Most visits to chiropractors and naturopathic physicians but less than one-third of visits to acupuncturists and massage therapists were covered by insurance.

The investigators commented on the observation that CAM providers typically did not discuss with the conventional doctors the care that they were providing to patients who were concurrently seeking care from conventional doctors. This finding, they argue, in conjunction with the fact that patients rarely discussed their CAM care with their conventional physicians raises concerns about the coordination and safety of concurrent care. A lack of coordination and safety issues are of particular concern when care is provided by acupuncturists and naturopathic physicians, who might prescribe herbs that interact with medication prescribed by conventional physicians and vice versa.

The investigators noted that although the overlap in the types of problems addressed by the four CAM professions is considerable, each profession has unique aspects. Chiropractors and massage therapists see the narrowest range of medical problems. However, chiropractors and massage therapists were the most likely to provide care not related to illness (e.g., care for wellness and prevention). Care for conditions other than illness in massage patients, which represented almost one in five visits, was focused on relaxation and stress reduction. Massage therapists also tend to see a substantial number of patients for self-reported anxiety or depression, some of whom might also want help relaxing and coping with stress. Another distinctive aspect of chiropractic care is the relatively large role that it plays in caring for acute conditions: about 40 percent of chiropractic visits are for acute conditions, whereas roughly 20 percent of visits to other CAM professionals are for acute conditions. As noted above, acupuncturists and naturopathic physicians see a broader range of conditions than chiropractors and massage therapists do and often provide care for such problems as anxiety, depression, fatigue, allergies, skin rashes, and menopausal symptoms.

The investigators commented that the most notable differences between the practices of conventional physicians (i.e., medical doctors and doctors of osteopathy) compared with those of CAM providers was the relatively large fraction of visits to the former for routine physical examinations, screening, and diagnostic tests and for symptoms associated with respiratory tract infections.

CONCLUSIONS AND RECOMMENDATIONS

As can be seen from the information presented in this chapter, an estimated 30 to 62 percent of adults in the United States use CAM. A lack of consensus on the definition of CAM has led to inconsistencies among the reports of various surveys on CAM prevalence and patterns of use. Total out-of-pocket expenditures for CAM therapies were conservatively estimated to be $27.0 billion in 1997. This is comparable to the projected out-of-pocket expenditures for all U.S. physician services (Eisenberg et al., 1998). The majority of CAM use is not reimbursed by insurance at present; however, data indicate that prevalence rates are likely to increase as third-party reimbursements for CAM benefits become increasingly available (Eisenberg et al., 1998; Wolsko et al., 2002). High-frequency users of CAM tend to be high-frequency users of health care in general and account for approximately 80 percent of the total expenditures on CAM. Many appear to use CAM for wellness and not just the treatment of disease (Wolsko et al., 2002). Women tend to use CAM more than men, and educated individuals tend to use CAM more than poorly educated individuals (Eisenberg et al., 1998; Wootton and Sparber, 2001a). However, CAM use is common among people in all ethnic groups (Barnes et al., 2004; Eisenberg et al., 1998; Mackenzie et al., 2003; Ni et al., 2002).

Although Eisenberg et al. (1993) and Wolsko et al. (2002) did find that a significant percentage of CAM use is unsupervised and engaged in as self-care, existing surveys reveal little about what percentage of CAM use is self-initiated ("I go to a provider and ask for X"), provider initiated ("I go to a provider, and she recommends or administers X"), provider administered ("She does X to me [massage, acupuncture, chiropractic]), or self-administered ("I read how to do it or someone shows me, and then I do it myself in a fashion I find comfortable; I self-regulate herbs, etc.)." Furthermore, few data are available on how the American public makes decisions about accessing CAM therapies. Finally, although there is an extensive literature on adherence to conventional treatment, there are virtually no data on rates of adherence to CAM treatment or self-treatment with CAM. This information is crucial to assessments of the real-world effectiveness and safety of CAM use.

A majority of patients who use CAM do not disclose such use to their physicians. Nondisclosure raises important safety issues, for example, the potential interactions of medications with herbs used as part of a CAM therapy. In addition, a majority of adults who use CAM therapies use more than one CAM modality and do so in combination with conventional medical care (Wolsko et al., 2002). Most adults who use both conventional and CAM therapies tend to value both for different purposes (Druss and Rosenheck, 1999; Eisenberg et al., 2001). Additionally, given the high rates of use of both CAM and conventional medicine by those with chronic conditions, there is a need for a better understanding of what motivates patients with such conditions to seek both CAM and conventional medical services and the cost implications of combined care.

The motivations for using CAM are numerous and are poorly captured by large-scale surveys; however, a major contributor appears to be the pursuit of wellness (Astin, 1998; Kessler et al., 2001; Wolsko et al., 2002). The extent to which CAM use is a trigger for positive behavioral change is unknown, however, and constitutes an important research issue because of the benefit of positive behavioral change to the public's health and its use as a means to address the escalating costs of health care. Longitudinal cohort studies can clarify people's trajectories of CAM use and those factors that influence upward and downward rates of use. Research designs that enable examination of patterns of CAM use need to be developed, as the patterns of CAM use are affected by external variables and influence other patterns of behavior important for health (e.g., diet, exercise, and substance use). Studies similar in structure to the Framingham Heart Study or the Nurses' Health Study (both of which are ongoing and which could be expanded to include questions about CAM) may offer the best opportunity to explore the patterns of CAM use over time and the role of CAM (or lack thereof) in promoting health, reducing risk, and preventing disease.

There is also little research on how the public obtains information about CAM modalities; what types of information are deemed credible, marginal, and spurious; how the public understands the information in terms of risks and benefits and how such perceptions inform decision making; and what the public expects providers to tell them. The few small studies that do exist illustrate that considerable misinformation is dispersed by vendors and on the Internet (Ashar et al., 2003; Bonakdar, 2002; Glisson et al., 2003; Matthews et al., 2003; Mills et al., 2003; Morris and Avorn, 2003). It is important to understand more about how the public is accessing information and making decisions about CAM use to move toward informed decision making about such therapies. Furthermore, closer monitoring of websites, enforcement of DSHEA and Federal Trade Commission regulations, and the creation of a user-friendly authoritative website on CAM modalities are needed.

As a means to address the lack of information discussed above, **the committee recommends that the National Institutes of Health and other public or private agencies sponsor quantitative and qualitative research to examine**

* **The social and cultural dimensions of illness experiences, health care-seeking processes and preferences, and practitioner-patient interaction;**
* **How often users of CAM, including patients and providers, adhere to treatment instructions and guidelines;**
* **The effects of CAM on wellness and disease prevention;**
* **How the American public accesses and evaluates information about CAM modalities; and**
* **Adverse events associated with CAM therapies and interactions between CAM and conventional treatments.**

Periodic surveys, especially in-depth instruments, would allow assessment of aspects of CAM prevalence, cost, and patterns of use that would not otherwise be captured by sentinel surveillance sites or ongoing, federally funded surveys. As discussed throughout this chapter we have little information about many aspects of CAM use. Surveys could, for example, provide much needed information about out-of-pocket costs and insured coverage for individual therapies; about the ingestion of individual prescription drugs, over-the-counter preparations, herbs, and supplements; the frequency of disclosure to one's doctor, nurse, pharmacist, or CAM provider about use of CAM therapies and the reasons for nondisclosure; and compliance issues including whether or to what extent use of CAM interferes with compliance with conventional treatments. Surveys could explore in depth the motivations for using CAM and investigate perceptions about various CAM therapies (and therapists) as compared with conventional therapies or therapists, stratified by disease, complaint, or CAM modality. Surveys are needed to provide information about how people obtain information about CAM; to investigate the impact of one person's CAM involvement on that person's immediate family or larger social network; and the impact of direct advertising to the public or the influence of CAM therapists and retailers of CAM products.

Further, **the committee recommends that the National Library of Medicine and other federal agencies develop criteria to assess the quality and reliability of information about CAM.**

When implementing the above recommendation regarding information about CAM, available criteria for assessment of health information in general should be examined and the applicability (or lack thereof) of existing criteria to CAM should be evaluated.

REFERENCES

Adler SR. 1999. Complementary and alternative medicine use among women with breast cancer. *Med Anthropol Q* 13(2):214–222.

Allaire AD, Moos MK, Wells SR. 2000. Complementary and alternative medicine in pregnancy: A survey of North Carolina certified nurse-midwives. *Obstet Gynecol* 95(1): 19–23.

Arora NK. 2003. Interacting with cancer patients: The significance of physicians' communication behavior. *Soc Sci Med* 57(5):791–806.

Ashar BH, Miller RG, Getz KJ, Pichard CP. 2003. A critical evaluation of Internet marketing of products that contain ephedra. *Mayo Clin Proc* 78(8):944–946.

Astin JA. 1998. Why patients use alternative medicine: Results of a national study. *JAMA* 279(19):1548–1553.

Astin JA, Pelletier KR, Marie A, Haskell WL. 2000. Complementary and alternative medicine use among elderly persons: One-year analysis of a Blue Shield Medicare supplement. *J Gerontol A Biol Sci Med Sci* 55(1):M4–M9.

Bair YA, Gold EB, Greendale GA, Sternfeld B, Adler SR, Azari R, Harkey M. 2002. Ethnic differences in use of complementary and alternative medicine at midlife: Longitudinal results from SWAN participants. *Am J Public Health* 92(11):1832–1840.

Barnes PM, Powell-Griner E, McFann K, Nahin RL. 2004. Complementary and alternative medicine use among adults: United States, 2002. *Vital Health and Statistics* 343:1–19 (advance data).

Baruch GK, Biener L, Barnett RC. 1987. Women and gender in research on work and family stress. *Am Psychol* 42(2):130–136.

Beal MW. 1998. Women's use of complementary and alternative therapies in reproductive health care. *J Nurse Midwifery* 43(3):224–234.

Bernstein BJ, Grasso T. 2001. Prevalence of complementary and alternative medicine use in cancer patients. *Oncology (Huntington)* 15(10):1267–1272.

Bertakis KD, Azari R, Helms LJ, Callahan EJ, Robbins JA. 2000. Gender differences in the utilization of health care services. *J Fam Pract* 49(2):147–152.

Bonakdar RA. 2002. Herbal cancer cures on the Web: Noncompliance with the Dietary Supplement Health and Education Act. *Fam Med* 34(7):522–527.

Braganza S, Ozuah PO, Sharif I. 2003. The use of complementary therapies in inner-city asthmatic children. *J Asthma* 40(7):823–827.

Breuner CC, Barry PJ, Kemper KJ. 1998. Alternative medicine use by homeless youth. *Arch Pediatr Adolesc Med* 152(11):1071–1075.

Burstein HJ, Gelber S, Guadagnoli E, Weeks JC. 1999. Use of alternative medicine by women with early-stage breast cancer. *N Engl J Med* 340(22):1733–1739.

Calder J, Issenman R, Cawdron R. 2000. Health information provided by retail health food outlets. *Can J Gastroenterol* 14(9):767–771.

Carpenter ES. 1980. Children's health care and the changing role of women. *Med Care* 18(12):1208–1218.

Chan E, Rappaport LA, Kemper KJ. 2003. Complementary and alternative therapies in childhood attention and hyperactivity problems. *J Dev Behav Pediatr* 24(1):4–8.

Cherkin DC, Eisenberg D, Sherman KJ, Barlow W, Kaptchuk TJ, Street J, Deyo RA. 2001. Randomized trial comparing traditional Chinese medical acupuncture, therapeutic massage, and self-care education for chronic low back pain. *Arch Intern Med* 161(8):1081–1088.

Cherkin DC, Deyo RA, Sherman KJ, Hart LG, Street JH, Hrbek A, Cramer E, Milliman B, Booker J, Mootz R, Barassi J, Kahn JR, Kaptchuk TJ, Eisenberg DM. 2002a. Characteristics of licensed acupuncturists, chiropractors, massage therapists, and naturopathic physicians. *J Am Board Fam Pract* 15(5):378–390.

Cherkin DC, Deyo RA, Sherman KJ, Hart LG, Street JH, Hrbek A, Davis RB, Cramer E, Milliman B, Booker J, Mootz R, Barassi J, Kahn JR, Kaptchuk TJ, Eisenberg DM. 2002b. Characteristics of visits to licensed acupuncturists, chiropractors, massage therapists, and naturopathic physicians. *J Am Board Fam Pract* 15(6):463–472.

Cherrington A, Lewis CE, McCreath HE, Herman CJ, Richter DL, Byrd T. 2003. Association of complementary and alternative medicine use, demographic factors, and perimenopausal symptoms in a multiethnic sample of women: The ENDOW study. *Fam Community Health* 26(1):74–83.

Clark L. 1995. Maternal responsibility for health in the household. *Health Care Wom Int* 16:43–55.

Cushman LF, Wade C, Factor-Litvak P, Kronenberg F, Firester L. 1999. Use of complementary and alternative medicine among African-American and Hispanic women in New York City: A pilot study. *J Am Med Womens Assoc* 54(4):193–195.

Davis MP, Darden PM. 2003. Use of complementary and alternative medicine by children in the United States. *Arch Pediatr Adolesc Med* 157(4):393–396.

DHHS (U.S. Department of Health and Human Services). 2000. *Healthy People 2010.* Washington, DC: U.S. Department of Health and Human Services.

DiMatteo MR, Giordani PJ, Lepper HS, Croghan TW. 2002. Patient adherence and medical treatment outcomes: A meta-analysis. *Med Care* 40(9):794–811.

Donovan JL, Blake DR. 1992. Patient non-compliance: Deviance or reasoned decision-making? *Soc Sci Med* 34(5):507–513.

Druss BG, Rosenheck RA. 1999. Association between use of unconventional therapies and conventional medical services. *JAMA* 282(7):651–656.

Druss BG, Marcus SC, Olfson M, Tanielian T, Elinson L, Pincus HA. 2001. Comparing the national economic burden of five chronic conditions. *Health Affairs (Millwood)* 20(6):233–241.

Easthope G. 1986. *Healers and Alternative Medicine: A Sociological Examination.* Brookfield, VT: Gower Publishing Company.

Easthope G, Tranter B, Gill G. 2000. General practitioners' attitudes toward complementary therapies. *Soc Sci Med* 51(10):1555–1561.

Eisenberg DM, Kessler RC, Foster C, Norlock FE, Calkins DR, Delbanco TL. 1993. Unconventional medicine in the United States. Prevalence, costs, and patterns of use. *N Engl J Med* 328(4):246–252.

Eisenberg DM, Davis RB, Ettner SL, Appel S, Wilkey S, Van Rompay M, Kessler RC. 1998. Trends in alternative medicine use in the United States, 1990-1997: Results of a follow-up national survey. *JAMA* 280(18):1569–1575.

Eisenberg DM, Kessler RC, Van Rompay MI, Kaptchuk TJ, Wilkey SA, Appel S, Davis RB. 2001. Perceptions about complementary therapies relative to conventional therapies among adults who use both: Results from a national survey. *Ann Intern Med* 135(5):344–351.

Factor-Litvak P, Cushman LF, Kronenberg F, Wade C, Kalmuss D. 2001. Use of complementary and alternative medicine among women in New York City: A pilot study. *J Altern Complement Med* 7(6):659–666.

Fairfield KM, Eisenberg DM, Davis RB, Libman H, Phillips RS. 1998. Patterns of use, expenditures, and perceived efficacy of complementary and alternative therapies in HIV-infected patients. *Arch Intern Med* 158(20):2257–2264.

Foote-Ardah CE. 2003. The meaning of complementary and alternative medicine practices among people with HIV in the United States: Strategies for managing everyday life. *Soc Health Ill* 25(5):481–500.

Foster DF, Phillips RS, Hamel MB, Eisenberg DM. 2000. Alternative medicine use in older Americans. *J Am Geriatr Soc* 48(12):1560–1565.

Fox S. 2002. *How Californians Compare to the Rest of the Nation.* A case study sponsored by the California Healthcare Foundation. Washington, DC: Pew Internet & American Life Project.

Fox S, Rainie L. 2002. *Vital Decisions: How Internet Users Decide What Information to Trust When They or Their Loved Ones Are Sick.* Washington, DC: Pew Internet & American Life Project.

Furnham A, Forey J. 1994. The attitudes, behaviors and beliefs of patients of conventional vs. complementary (alternative) medicine. *J Clin Psychol* 50(3):458–469.

Furnham A, Smith C. 1988. Choosing alternative medicine: A comparison of the beliefs of patients visiting a general practitioner and a homoeopath. *Soc Sci Med* 26(7):685–689.

Gijsbers van Wijk CM, Kolk AM, van den Bosch WJ, van den Hoogen HJ. 1992. Male and female morbidity in general practice: The nature of sex differences. *Soc Sci Med* 35(5): 665–678.

Glisson JK, Rogers HE, Abourashed EA, Ogletree R, Hufford CD, Khan I. 2003. Clinic at the health food store? Employee recommendations and product analysis. *Pharmacotherapy* 23(1):64–72.

Gordon NP, Sobel DS, Tarazona EZ. 1998. Use of and interest in alternative therapies among adult primary care clinicians and adult members in a large health maintenance organization. *West J Med* 169(3):153–161.

Greendale GA, Young JT, Huang MH, Bucur A, Want Y, Seeman T. 2003. Hip axis length in mid-life Japanese and Caucasian vs. residents: No evidence for an ethnic difference. *Osteoporosis Int* 14:320–325.

Gulla J, Singer AJ. 2000. Use of alternative therapies among emergency department patients. *Ann Emerg Med* 35(3):226–228.

Henderson JW, Donatelle RJ. 2004. Complementary and alternative medicine use by women after completion of allopathic treatment for breast cancer. *Altern Ther Health Med* 10(1):52–57.

Hepner DL, Harnett M, Segal S, Camann W, Bader AM, Tsen LC. 2002. Herbal medicine use in parturients. *Anesth Analg* 94(3):690–693.

Hibbard JH, Pope CR. 1983. Gender roles, illness orientation and use of medical services. *Soc Sci Med* 17(3):129–137.

Hoffman C, Rice D, Sung HY. 1996. Persons with chronic conditions. Their prevalence and costs. *JAMA* 276(18):1473–1479.

Kaplan RM. 1988. Health-related quality of life with applicatons in nutrition research and practice. *Clin Nutr* 7:64–70.

Kao GD, Devine P. 2000. Use of complementary health practices by prostate carcinoma patients undergoing radiation therapy. *Cancer* 88(3):615–619.

Kaptchuk TJ, Eisenberg DM. 1998. The persuasive appeal of alternative medicine. *Ann Intern Med* 129(12):1061–1065.

Kelner M, Wellman B. 1997. Health care and consumer choice: Medical and alternative therapies. *Soc Sci Med* 45(2):203–212.

Kessler RC, Davis RB, Foster DF, Van Rompay MI, Walters EE, Wilkey SA, Kaptchuk TJ, Eisenberg DM. 2001. Long-term trends in the use of complementary and alternative medical therapies in the United States. *Ann Intern Med* 135(4):262–268.

Kitai E, Vinker S, Sandiuk A, Hornik O, Zeltcer C, Gaver A. 1998. Use of complementary and alternative medicine among primary care patients. *Fam Pract* 15(5):411–414.

Korthals-de Bos IB, Hoving JL, van Tulder MW, Rutten-van Molken MP, Ader HJ, de Vet HC, Koes BW, Vondeling H, Bouter LM. 2003. Cost effectiveness of physiotherapy, manual therapy, and general practitioner care for neck pain: Economic evaluation alongside a randomised controlled trial. *BMJ* 326(7395):911.

Krauss HH, Godfrey C, Kirk J, Eisenberg DM. 1998. Alternative health care: Its use by individuals with physical disabilities. *Arch Phys Med Rehabil* 79(11):1440–1447.

Kronenberg F, Fugh-Berman A. 2002. Complementary and alternative medicine for menopausal symptoms: A review of randomized, controlled trials. *Ann Intern Med* 137(10):805–813.

Krouse JH, Krouse HJ. 1999. Patient use of traditional and complementary therapies in treating rhinosinusitis before consulting an otolaryngologist. *Laryngoscope* 109(8):1223–1227.

Lee AC, Li DH, Kemper KJ. 2000a. Chiropractic care for children. *Arch Pediatr Adolesc Med* 154(4):401–407.

Lee MM, Lin SS, Wrensch MR, Adler SR, Eisenberg D. 2000b. Alternative therapies used by women with breast cancer in four ethnic populations. *J Natl Cancer Inst* 92(1):42–47.

Lee MM, Chang JS, Jacobs B, Wrensch MR. 2002. Complementary and alternative medicine use among men with prostate cancer in 4 ethnic populations. *Am J Public Health* 92(10):1606–1609.

Lengacher CA, Bennett MP, Kip KE, Keller R, LaVance MS, Smith LS, Cox CE. 2002. Frequency of use of complementary and alternative medicine in women with breast cancer. *Oncol Nurs Forum* 29(10):1445–1452.

Lloyd P, Lupton D, Wiesner D, Hasleton S. 1993. Choosing alternative therapy: An exploratory study of sociodemographic characteristics and motives of patients resident in Sydney. *Aust J Public Health* 17(2):135–144.

Macintyre S, Hunt K, Sweeting H. 1996. Gender differences in health: Are things really as simple as they seem? *Soc Sci Med* 42(4):617–624.

Mackenzie ER, Taylor L, Bloom BS, Hufford DJ, Johnson JC. 2003. Ethnic minority use of complementary and alternative medicine (CAM): A national probability survey of CAM utilizers. *Altern Ther Health Med* 9(4):50–56.

Madsen H, Andersen S, Nielsen RG, Dolmer BS, Host A, Damkier A. 2003. Use of complementary/alternative medicine among paediatric patients. *Eur J Pediatr* 162(5):334–341.

Maskarinec G, Shumay DM, Kakai H, Gotay CC. 2000. Ethnic differences in complementary and alternative medicine use among cancer patients. *J Altern Complement Med* 6(6):531–538.

Matthews SC, Camacho A, Mills PJ, Dimsdale JE. 2003. The Internet for medical information about cancer: Help or hindrance? *Psychosomatics* 44(2):100–103.

Michelson W. 1990. Child care and the daily routine. *Social Indicators Research* 23:353–366.

Mills E, Ernst E, Singh R, Ross C, Wilson K. 2003. Health food store recommendations: Implications for breast cancer patients. *Breast Cancer Res* 5(6):R170–R174.

Mitchell A, Cormack MA. 1998. *The Therapeutic Relationship in Complementary Health Care*. Edinburgh: Churchill Livingstone Press.

Morris CA, Avorn J. 2003. Internet marketing of herbal products. *JAMA* 290(11):1505–1509.

Mustard CA, Kaufert P, Kozyrskyj A, Mayer T. 1998. Sex differences in the use of health care services. *N Engl J Med* 338(23):1678–1683.

Najm W, Reinsch S, Hoehler F, Tobis J. 2003. Use of complementary and alternative medicine among the ethnic elderly. *Altern Ther Health Med* 9(3):50–57.

Ni H, Simile C, Hardy AM. 2002. Utilization of complementary and alternative medicine by United States adults: Results from the 1999 National Health Interview Survey. *Med Care* 40(4):353–358.

Nichter M. 2003. Harm reduction: A core concern for medical anthropology. In: Harthorn BH, Oaks L, eds. *Risk, Culture, and Health Inequality: Shifting Perceptions of Danger and Blame*. Westport, CT: Praeger Press.

Norred CL, Zamudio S, Palmer SK. 2000. Use of complementary and alternative medicines by surgical patients. *AANA J* 68(1):13–18.

Paramore LC. 1997. Use of alternative therapies: Estimates from the 1994 Robert Wood Johnson Foundation National Access to Care Survey. *J Pain Symptom Management* 13(2):83–89.

Patterson RE, Neuhouser ML, Hedderson MM, Schwartz SM, Standish LJ, Bowen DJ, Marshall LM. 2002. Types of alternative medicine used by patients with breast, colon, or prostate cancer: Predictors, motives, and costs. *J Altern Complement Med* 8(4):4 77–485.

Pawluch D, Cain R, Gillett J. 2000. Lay constructions of HIV and complementary therapy use. *Soc Sci Med* 51(2):251–264.

Rao JK, Mihaliak K, Kroenke K, Bradley J, Tierney WM, Weinberger M. 1999. Use of complementary therapies for arthritis among patients of rheumatologists. *Ann Intern Med* 131(6):409–416.

Rawsthorne P, Shanahan F, Cronin NC, Anton PA, Lofberg R, Bohman L, Bernstein CN. 1999. An international survey of the use and attitudes regarding alternative medicine by patients with inflammatory bowel disease. *Am J Gastroenterol* 94(5):1298–1303.

Richardson MA, Sanders T, Palmer JL, Greisinger A, Singletary SE. 2000. Complementary/alternative medicine use in a comprehensive cancer center and the implications for oncology. *J Clin Oncol* 18(13):2505–2514.

Rogers EA, Gough JE, Brewer KL. 2001. Are emergency department patients at risk for herb-drug interactions? *Acad Emerg Med* 8(9):932–934.

Sagaram S, Walji M, Bernstam E. 2002. Evaluating the prevalence, content and readability of complementary and alternative medicine (CAM) web pages on the internet. *Proc AMIA Symp*. Pp. 672–676.

Sawni-Sikand A, Schubiner H, Thomas RL. 2002. Use of complementary/alternative therapies among children in primary care pediatrics. *Ambul Pediatr* 2(2):99–103.

Sharma U. 1992. *Complementary Medicine Today: Practitioners and Patients*. New York: Tavistock/Routledge.

Sharma U. 1993. Contextualizing alternative medicine. The exotic, the marginal and the perfectly mundane. *Anthropol Today* 9(4):15–18.

Sharma U. 1996. Using complementary therapies: A challenge to orthodox medicine? In: Williams SJ, Calnan M, eds. *Modern Medicine: Lay Perspectives and Experiences*. London: UCL Press. Pp. 230–255.

Siahpush M. 1999. Why do people favour alternative medicine? *Aust N Z J Public Health* 23(3):266–271.

Sirois FM. 2002. Treatment seeking and experience with complementary/alternative medicine: A continuum of choice. *J Altern Complement Med* 8(2):127–134.

Sirois FM, Gick ML. 2002. An investigation of the health beliefs and motivations of complementary medicine clients. *Soc Sci Med* 55(6):1025–1037.

Sobel DS. 2000. MSJAMA: Mind matters, money matters: the cost-effectiveness of mind/body medicine. *JAMA* 284(13):1705.

Sollner W, Maislinger S, DeVries A, Steixner E, Rumpold G, Lukas P. 2000. Use of complementary and alternative medicine by cancer patients is not associated with perceived distress or poor compliance with standard treatment but with active coping behavior: A survey. *Cancer* 89(4):873–880.

Sparber A, Wootton JC. 2001. Surveys of complementary and alternative medicine. Part II. Use of alternative and complementary cancer therapies. *J Altern Complement Med* 7(3):281–287.

Sparber A, Wootton JC. 2002. Surveys of complementary and alternative medicine. Part V. Use of alternative and complementary therapies for psychiatric and neurologic diseases. *J Altern Complement Med* 8(1):93–96.

Sparber A, Bauer L, Curt G, Eisenberg D, Levin T, Parks S, Steinberg SM, Wootton J. 2000. Use of complementary medicine by adult patients participating in cancer clinical trials. *Oncol Nurs Forum* 27(4):623–630.

Stanger J, Couglan B. 2000. Complementary and alternative medicine: What employers need to know. *Compensation & Benefits Management* 16(1):1–8.

Swisher EM, Cohn DE, Goff BA, Parham J, Herzog TJ, Rader JS, Mutch DG. 2002. Use of complementary and alternative medicine among women with gynecologic cancers. *Gynecol Oncol* 84(3):363–367.

Thorne S, Paterson B, Russell C, Schultz A. 2002. Complementary/alternative medicine in chronic illness as informed self-care decision making. *Int J Nurs Studies* 39(7):671–683.

Tillman R. 2002. Paying for alternative medicine: The role of health insurers. *Ann Am Acad Polit Soc Sci* 583:64–75.

Tiran D. 2002. Nausea and vomiting in pregnancy: Safety and efficacy of self-administered complementary therapies. *Complement Ther Nurs Midwifery* 8(4):191–196.

Umberson D. 1992. Gender, marital status and the social control of health behavior. *Soc Sci Med* 34(8):907–917.

Vallerand AH, Fouladbakhsh JM, Templin T. 2003. The use of complementary/alternative medicine therapies for the self-treatment of pain among residents of urban, suburban, and rural communities. *Am J Public Health* 93(6):923–925.

VandeCreek L, Rogers E, Lester J. 1999. Use of alternative therapies among breast cancer outpatients compared with the general population. *Altern Ther Health Med* 5(1):71–76.

Verbrugge LM. 1989. The twain meet: Empirical explanations of sex differences in health and mortality. *J Health Soc Behav* 30(3):282–304.

Verbrugge LM, Wingard DL. 1987. Sex differentials in health and mortality. *Women Health* 12(2):103–145. Rec #:615.

Vermeire E, Hearnshaw H, Van Royen P, Denekens J. 2001. Patient adherence to treatment: Three decades of research. A comprehensive review. *J Clin Pharm Ther* 26(5):331–342.

Von Gruenigen VE, White LJ, Kirven MS, Showalter AL, Hopkins MP, Jenison EL. 2001. A comparison of complementary and alternative medicine use by gynecology and gynecologic oncology patients. *Int J Gynecol Cancer* 11(3):205–209.

Weiss SJ, Takakuwa KM, Ernst AA. 2001. Use, understanding, and beliefs about complementary and alternative medicines among emergency department patients. *Acad Emerg Med* 8(1):41–47.

White AR, Ernst E. 2000. Economic analysis of complementary medicine: A systematic review. *Complement Ther Med* 8(2):111–118.

Wilkinson S, Gomella LG, Smith JA, Brawer MK, Dawson NA, Wajsman Z, Dai L, Chodak GW. 2002. Attitudes and use of complementary medicine in men with prostate cancer. *J Urol* 168(6):2505–2509.

Wolsko PM, Eisenberg DM, Davis RB, Ettner SL, Phillips RS. 2002. Insurance coverage, medical conditions, and visits to alternative medicine providers: Results of a national survey. *Arch Intern Med* 162(3):281–287.

Wonderling D, Vickers AJ, Grieve R, McCarney R. 2004. Cost effectiveness analysis of a randomised trial of acupuncture for chronic headache in primary care. *BMJ* 328(7442):747.

Wootton JC, Sparber A. 2001a. Surveys of complementary and alternative medicine. Part I. General trends and demographic groups. *J Altern Complement Med* 7(2):195–208.

Wootton JC, Sparber A. 2001b. Surveys of complementary and alternative medicine. Part III. Use of alternative and complementary therapies for HIV/AIDS. *J Altern Complement Med* 7(4):371–377.

Wootton JC, Sparber A. 2001c. Surveys of complementary and alternative medicine. Part IV. Use of alternative and complementary therapies for rheumatologic and other diseases. *J Altern Complement Med* 7(6):715–721.

Zimmerman RA, Thompson IM Jr. 2002. Prevalence of complementary medicine in urologic practice. A review of recent studies with emphasis on use among prostate cancer patients. *Urol Clin N Am* 29(1):vii, 1–9.

3

Contemporary Approaches to Evidence of Treatment Effectiveness: A Context for CAM Research

Evidence of treatment effectiveness from clinical research has become integral to effective clinical care. This chapter provides a context for the committee's recommendations about research on complementary and alternative medicine (CAM) that appear in Chapters 4 and 5. A brief account of the development of present approaches to evidence-driven clinical and public policy (which includes practice guidelines and coverage policy) is presented. This is followed by a description of the basic ideas of clinical research design, including a taxonomy of study design and a taxonomy of outcome measurements. An account of some features of contemporary data analysis follows. The chapter concludes with an overview of the applicability of contemporary clinical research methods to some CAM therapies.

A BRIEF ACCOUNT OF THE DEVELOPMENT OF TREATMENT EFFECTIVENESS RESEARCH

As noted in Chapter 1, over the past twenty years practitioners of conventional medicine have made a marked shift from a reliance on experience (directly observed or as recorded by others in medical journals) to a reliance on more rigorous research to evaluate the effectiveness of treatments. For example, the concept of formal evaluation of therapies through randomized controlled trials is certainly not new (Kaptchuk and Kerr, 2004) but has regularly been applied in Western medicine only since World War II (Byar, 1980; Cochrane, 1972).

Some notable exceptions to reliance on experience exist, however. In the middle of the nineteenth century, Florence Nightingale pioneered the application of epidemiological and statistical methods to the study of hospital deaths, and her discoveries of a plausible causal relationship between processes of care and outcomes led to challenges to thoughts about mechanisms of disease prevalent at the time, changes in clinical practice, and improvements in mortality rates. In the early twentieth century, Ernest Amory Codman, a Boston surgeon, argued strongly for the formal study of surgical outcomes in an effort to understand which surgeons, hospitals, and surgical procedures produced good versus bad outcomes (Neuhauser, 2002). This effort did not take root and grow—in fact, it provoked significant hostility among Codman's colleagues—but it raised the question of the need for formal analysis of treatment outcomes that was picked up again more than 50 years later.

The need for formal evidence of effectiveness for common medical and surgical interventions was recognized much more broadly beginning in the 1970s. Passage of Medicare and Medicaid legislation, together with apparent advances in medical and surgical care, contributed to a surge in health care spending. Policy makers and payers asked increasingly pointed questions about the "value" of health care, questions that required more fundamental questions about the effectiveness of interventions to be answered.

Even more disquieting questions emerged from a body of work that described striking variations in the rates of common surgical procedures such as surgery for benign prostate disease, hysterectomy, and tonsillectomy, among seemingly similar geographic regions. This work began in the late 1960s in northern New England, where isolated hospital market areas could easily be defined (Wennberg and Gittelsohn, 1982).

International differences in the rates of medical procedures were observed; and when the variations *within* countries were adjusted for the overall rate of variation *among* countries, a consistent pattern was detected; a high degree of variation was a marker for a high degree of discretion, and a high degree of discretion was often explained by professional uncertainty about effectiveness (McPherson et al., 1982). At the time, few of the procedures in question had been subjected to randomized controlled clinical trials or other credible clinical studies. Subsequently, variations in the rates of medical admission, physician visits, and diagnostic tests that could not be explained by clinical variables were also found. Taken together, these findings raised new questions about the science base of clinical practice. If decisions were based on science, how could it be that treatment depended more on where one lived than what was wrong or what one cared about? Policy makers wondered if high rates meant overuse and economic waste and if low rates meant underuse and deprivation. "Which rate was right?" became the pressing policy question and the answer required a new investment in clinical research to better define the outcomes of common interventions for common conditions. Thus, the practice variation phenomenon provided the motivation and the rationale for the development of "outcomes research."

The goal of outcomes research was to determine what was known and what was not known about common interventions, thereby setting research agendas for common conditions. Existing evidence was systematically reviewed by using techniques for combining data from different studies previously described in the social sciences. Claims data linked to Social Security Administration mortality and other administrative data were used to glean outcomes information to fill the gaps in knowledge that existed at the time. Patient surveys were conducted to capture patients' subjective responses to treatments and outcomes. Variations in these responses highlighted the importance of patients' preferences as a source of warranted variation in clinical decisions. Decision models (a model is a representation of reality) were constructed to test the relative sensitivities of decisions to key probabilities of good or bad outcomes and to patient preferences. Decision support tools were developed; and trials were designed to help patients and doctors choose among treatment options, including randomization in a trial when a well-informed patient was at equipoise, that is, finding each treatment equally acceptable.

Other investigators used consensus methods to develop appropriateness criteria that were then applied to the medical records of patients who had undergone procedures with high rates of variation by geographic region. It was common for procedures for 30 percent or more of patients' indications to be deemed inappropriate. The proportions of procedures deemed inappropriate was essentially the same in high- and low-volume settings, so the low-volume providers were not simply doing a better job of selecting only appropriate cases.

This work was extended with a focus on guideline development. Professional organizations such as the American College of Physicians instituted rigorous guideline development processes, increasing recognition of the severe limitations of the evidence base for the treatment of common conditions.

Evidence of Effectiveness for Prescription Drugs

The limited evidence base for surgery and other procedures for the common conditions targeted by outcomes research contrasted sharply with the richer body of evidence for medical therapies. This difference can best be understood in the context of the regulation of medications that began in 1906 with the Pure Food and Drug Act, which made misrepresentation of ingredients illegal and which recognized the standardized drug formulae registered in a national formulary or pharmacopoeia. The 1906 act was silent on drug safety and efficacy.

The Federal Food, Drug, and Cosmetic Act of 1938 extended safeguards by introducing the distinction between prescription and over-the-counter drugs and requiring pharmaceutical manufacturers to prove drug safety information before the drug could be released for use. This was a direct response to the elixir sulfanilamide tragedy, in which 107 people, most of them children, died when a new sulfa preparation was distributed without testing of the preparation for safety.

In 1951, the Durham-Humphrey Amendment (U.S. Statutes at Large, 1951) made it clear that the classification of drugs as prescription was up to the Food and Drug Administration (FDA), not manufacturers. In its initial form, the amendment authorized FDA to test drugs for efficacy as well as safety. However, the efficacy requirement was eventually removed before passage of the amendment. The next significant change in legislation followed the thalidomide disaster in Europe, which was narrowly averted in the United States and which prompted passage of the Kefauver-Harris Amendment (U.S. Statutes at Large, 1962) in 1962. All clinical testing procedures had to be approved by FDA and had to demonstrate efficacy as well as safety. The pharmaceutical industry resisted the efficacy requirement, especially the retroactive evaluation of drugs. However, in 1970, in the court case *Upjohn Co. v. Finch* (422 F.2d 944, 955 [6th Cir. 1970]), the Court of Appeals ruled that commercial success alone did not constitute substantial evidence for efficacy in the case of the Upjohn drug Panalba. Evidence of efficacy as well as of safety had become an enforceable standard for prescription drugs. Over the ensuing decades, the pharmaceutical industry and clinical research organizations (CROs[1]) rapidly built the capacity to conduct those clinical trials necessary to meet the standards set by FDA.

More Recent Developments: Evidence-Based Medicine

As the need for evidence became more evident and funding for clinical research became more available, many academic settings emphasized development and use of methods for gathering clinical evidence. The multidisciplinary collaborations that formed with federally funded "patient outcomes research teams" matured as methodological expertise in clinical epidemiology, decision theory, and other domains of quantitative and qualitative research was honed. The "clinimetrics" work of Alvan Feinstein at Yale attracted more attention. David Sackett and colleagues in Canada and

---

[1]CROs provide a wide range of research and development services. CROs assist pharmaceutical, biotechnology, and medical device companies to produce new medicines and new treatments (www.acrohealth.org).

later England defined clinical epidemiology as the "basic science for clinicians." Courses were devised to teach students and physicians how to critically appraise the medical literature. Fellowship and clinical scholar programs turned out clinical scientists with the skills necessary to generate and accurately interpret evidence. The Canadian Task Force on the Periodic Physical Examination and later the U.S. Preventive Services Task Force developed ratings for "levels of evidence," which are described in detail later in this chapter. The Cochrane Collaboration was formed in Oxford, England, to systematically examine evidence for the full breadth of medical practice and quickly attracted an extensive international following. Journals with the titles *Evidence-Based Medicine* and *Evidence-Based Health Care* appeared. By the mid-1990s, the concept of formal, scientific evidence of treatment effectiveness had arrived, at least in some circles.

The goal of evidence-based medicine is to ensure that, to the extent possible, individual clinical decisions and broader health policy decisions about tests and treatments be based on the published results of rigorous studies of efficacy and effectiveness. Because not all treatments have been subjected to formal study and because some treatments cannot be studied without investment in massive clinical trials, it will not be possible to base all treatment decisions on published evidence. Nevertheless, the concept of evidence-based medicine asks that decisions be based on published scientific evidence when it is available and that investments be made to gather evidence in as many areas of medical care as possible.

In conventional medicine, there is now a general acceptance of the need to carefully study the effectiveness of tests and treatments, even those that have already become frequently used. Just in the past 3 years, prominent studies have challenged the effectiveness of bone marrow transplantation and high-dose chemotherapy for breast cancer (Farquhar et al., 2003), arthroscopic surgery for osteoarthritis of the knee (Moseley et al., 2002), and the use of estrogen replacement therapy during menopause (Rossouw et al., 2002).

There are clearly *some* treatments for which evidence of effectiveness is immediate and compelling. It may be unnecessary or even unethical to conduct formal effectiveness trials in a variety of situations, for example, when a treatment results in a combination of a clear reversal or elimination of a disease process, has a short latency of noticeable effect, is nearly universally effective in all patients treated, and eliminates clinical symptoms. The use of penicillin in the mid-1940s, surgery for appendicitis, and resection of localized cancers all stand as examples of this sort of undisputed effectiveness. Even in these examples, there may be value in conducting long-term surveillance studies to detect rare or late complications or side effects, and it may be appropriate to conduct formal cost-effectiveness or cost-benefit studies.

At the other end of the spectrum are those interventions that have modest effects, if any at all. It is these interventions that require studies with rigorous design and of rigorous execution to determine whether an effect does indeed exist and to estimate its size.

The next section examines a variety of research methods available for use in conducting clinical effectiveness research.

BASIC FEATURES OF CONTEMPORARY CLINICAL EFFECTIVENESS RESEARCH

A Taxonomy of Clinical Research Methods

Many factors can influence the outcome of treatment. These include the treatment itself, characteristics of the patient (such as age, gender, and comorbid conditions), other treatments, access to care, adherence to treatment plans, socioeconomic status and education, and the skill of the practitioner. In treatment effectiveness research, the goal is to evaluate the contribution of one of these factors, treatment, to determine whether treatment makes a difference. Doing so can be difficult if other factors are at play, as they often are. The goal of study designs is usually to make it possible to assess the contribution of the treatment after the other influences on outcome are taken into account.

In a study comparing two clinical interventions, the goal is to be sure that any difference observed is due to the differences in the two interventions rather than some other factor. The "some other factor" is a "confounder," because it confounds one's efforts to draw the conclusion that differences between the interventions are responsible for the differences in outcomes.

Random Assignment to Treatment or Control

The best way to be sure that one can draw a strong conclusion from a difference in outcomes is to assign subjects randomly to receive one intervention or the other. If the randomization is successful and the number of patients is large enough, the two study populations will be essentially identical except for the different interventions. If one conducts the study so that, except for the intervention, the study populations are also identical at the end of the study, the researchers can make a very strong inference that the cause of the differences in outcomes is the difference in the interventions. Randomization is powerful because it ensures that the two populations are similar in every respect except for the intervention to which the researchers randomly assigned the patients. This claim means that if the study groups are large enough and the randomization was successful, the frequencies of all known factors (e.g., age, gender, and comorbid conditions) are similar in both groups; in addition, and perhaps more importantly, the frequency of any *unknown* or *unmeasured* factor will be the same in both groups. Randomized trials stand at the top of the hierarchy of evidence because they make it possible to infer a cause-and-effect relationship between an intervention and an outcome. Because the study groups are identical except for the intervention, any effect on outcomes must be due to the intervention.

Observational Studies

Other methods for studying the effects of two interventions rely on data derived from the observation of care. In contrast to a randomized trial, no one intervenes in an observational study. Instead, researchers use information about the patients to try to make inferences about the relationship of clinical factors (including treatment) to clinical outcomes. Sometimes, researchers collect the information systematically (a prospective study); other times, the data represent patient care as it happened in the past (retrospective study). In either case, the crucial distinguishing feature of an observational study is that receipt of the intervention depends on clinical circumstances and preferences rather than deliberate assignment, as in a randomized clinical trial. These circumstances that influence choice of treatment may also influence the outcomes. Differences in outcomes may therefore be due to the intervention *or* other circumstances, or a combination of both.

Observational studies have many advantages. They are much less costly than randomized trials, they can have huge study populations, and the results are more likely to represent practice (Benson and Hartz, 2000). However, the circumstances that influence the choice of treatment often *confound* the interpretation of differences in outcomes. The frequencies of potential confounders may differ between those who receive the intervention and those who do not. To evaluate differences in outcomes independently of the influence of possible confounders, researchers perform multivariable regression techniques on the data. The variables used in the statistical model are either the several candidate predictor variables (the treatment itself and other potential confounders, such as demographic characteristics, clinical characteristics of the patient, comorbid conditions, and socioeconomic factors) or the dependent variable (the outcome that the model is trying to predict). These techniques effectively adjust the frequencies of the confounders measured so that they occur at the same rate in both the treatment and the no-treatment groups. If the treatment is still a statistically significant predictor of an outcome, researchers can infer an association between the outcome and the treatment. However, they cannot infer that the treatment causes the outcome because the statistical techniques can only adjust for differences in the confounders that the researchers measured. Unmeasured confounders are thus the bane of researchers who conduct observational studies.

Therefore, the possibility that a confounding variable is responsible for observed differences means that one must express conclusions in terms of association rather than causation. Even then, researchers must be cautious in their conclusions because it is possible that the apparent association between two variables is actually the result of a third variable (the confounder) that is affecting the two variables at the same time so that they change in concert. In observational studies, the researchers must guard against concluding that the change in one variable is the consequence of the change in the other variable (cause and effect).

Types of Observational Studies Observational studies come in several forms: cohort studies, case-control studies, case series, and cross-sectional and longitudinal studies. Each of these is described below.

Cohort Studies. A cohort study (in the context of treatment effectiveness research) is the formal collection and analysis of data on treatments and outcomes for a defined set of patients with similar clinical characteristics. For example, a researcher might study pain and disability levels as outcomes in a cohort of patients older than 70 years of age who received lumbar fusion surgery for severe sciatica. The distinguishing feature of cohort studies is that researchers gather data on treatment and possible confounders at one point in time and measure outcomes at a later point in time. Cohort studies are a relatively powerful form of study design because researchers can often statistically adjust the final outcomes (e.g., levels of pain) for differences in the outcome variable at the beginning of the study (pain levels before surgery) and because they can measure the outcome variable at many points in time (e.g., from monthly pain reports for up to 2 years after surgery).

The assembly of a cohort is the first step. It may take place in the present as a deliberate, planned activity in which the researchers gather data on the present state of the participants (prospective cohort), or it may rely upon data gathered in the past (retrospective cohort). In either case, the investigators use specific inclusion and exclusion criteria to define a group of people with many similarities. Even though members of the cohort are similar in terms of the inclusion criteria (in the example cited above, all patients will be older than age 70 years, all will have had fusion surgery, and all will have had severe sciatica before surgery), they will inevitably differ in many other predictors of outcome. For example, some members of the spine surgery cohort may be 70 years old and others may be 85 years old. Some may be overweight and others may be thin. Some will be engaged in regularly physical activity, and others will be sedentary. Some will have a spouse or caregiver available to help with work at home; others will be on their own. All of these factors, and countless others, may have influences on treatment outcomes. Researchers try to identify and record as many of these factors as possible, but inevitably some potentially important factors are not measured.

Outcome measurement is the second major step. The researchers measure outcomes at a future time relative to the date of cohort assembly. With a prospective cohort, measurement of outcomes occurs in the future at specific time points relative to the date of treatment. With a retrospective cohort, the outcomes may have occurred in the past relative to the date of treatment and may have to be abstracted from existing data systems or may still occur in the future if members of the cohort are still alive and available for follow-up.

Case-Control Studies. The study population in a case-control study in the domain of treatment effectiveness consists of the cases (those with the target outcome, such as complete pain relief) and the controls (those without the target outcome, for example, those with continued pain). Case-control studies are especially well-suited to studies of rare events, because cases (those experiencing the event) are oversampled relative to the controls. Case-control studies are typically retrospective, in that the researchers assemble the study population after the measurable outcome events have occurred. If adequate numbers of patients are available, researchers choose the controls by matching each control patient (or several control patients) to one case patient for variables such as age, sex, and date of entry into the population from which the researchers identify cases and controls. The next step is to measure rates of exposure to a treatment (e.g., a surgical procedure) for the cases and the controls. The ratio of the rates of exposure to the intervention for those who experience the outcome (cases) and those who do not experience it (controls) is mathematically equivalent to the ratio of the outcomes in those exposed to the intervention to the rate in those not exposed to it. Thus, the outcome of a case-control study is a rate ratio or an odds ratio of the target condition frequency in exposed patients versus that in unexposed patients. Researchers may perform regression analysis techniques to adjust the cases and controls for differences in potential confounders. The Achilles heel of a case-control study is confounders, and the researchers' greatest challenge is assembling the control group to avoid confounders. One way to accomplish this task is to choose cases and controls from a cohort that the researchers assembled using the same inclusion and exclusion criteria (a so-called nested case-control study).

Case Series. A case series is simply a serial collection of patients with some defining characteristic. A typical case series is a group of patients who have a rare diagnosis or who have undergone a new surgical procedure. In the context of treatment effectiveness research, a case series would be a consecutive set of patients who received a particular treatment. Case series do not have controls, so that it is very difficult to make any inferences about whether an intervention (a treatment or surgical procedure) had any effect. An exception would have been the first group of patients with pneumonia who received penicillin and experienced rates of survival that were unprecedented in the era before penicillin. In surgical research, it is reasonably common to publish results of case series studies and to compare the outcomes to those for other published case series for patients with the same underlying condition. These "historical controls" provide a basis for comparison of outcomes for the new treatment, but it is even more difficult to draw inferences in a case series study than in either a prospective or a retrospective cohort study because the patients in the comparison group were treated at a different place and at a different time, so there are confounders related to place and time, in addition to the confounders in the cohort study related to the patients' clinical and personal characteristics.

Cross-Sectional and Longitudinal Studies. Cross-sectional studies measure the relationship between variables at a single point in time. Cross-sectional studies are a relatively weak study design for the testing of hypotheses about treatment-outcome relationships because they rely upon a single measurement of each variable. A survey is a typical cross-sectional study design. Longitudinal studies measure the relationship between variables at two or more points in time. In effectiveness studies, longitudinal studies would typically involve the measurement of outcomes at several points after treatment. They are a relatively powerful method for the testing of hypotheses because repeating a measurement many times (or even once) for an individual reduces statistical variation and narrows confidence intervals.

Clinical Outcomes: A Taxonomy

Treatment outcomes can be objective or subjective. Objective outcomes are visible or measurable to people other than the patient, and subjective outcomes can be felt or reported only by the patient. One of the major contributions of the outcomes management movement in the late 1980s and early 1990s was to raise the status of subjective measures as valid scientific endpoints in clinical trials and other forms of research studies. Advances in the technology of subjective measurement made that change possible, so that it is now common to find a mix of subjective and objective endpoints in many clinical trials.

Subjective Outcomes

Subjective outcomes include those symptoms and other aspects of a patient's experience that are not directly observable by others, but that represent the goals of treatment. Pain, sensations of nausea or dizziness, functional status, ability to perform activities of daily living, and experience of moods or emotional states are examples of subjective outcomes for which well-developed and widely used measures exist (Bowling, 1997; Frank-Stromborg and Olsen, 1997; McDowell and Newell, 1996). Because there is no direct way to validate a patient's report of pain level or mood state, the development of valid measures requires careful attention to issues of reliability (i.e., whether measures taken at two adjacent points in time yield the same result or whether two closely related versions of the same scale yield the same result) and convergent validity (i.e., whether the results of two presumably related, but different, measures actually yield similar results). Because patients' responses to single questions or item formats may be affected by idiosyncrasies of wording and interpretation, it is common for measures of subjective outcomes to be based on multi-item scales with different wordings and response formats. Patient reports may also be sensitive to context or contrast effects (for example, a relatively modest "absolute" level of pain may feel uncomfortable if it is new but may feel very minor if it has been preceded by a long period of excruciating, severe pain).

The subjective domains for which well-established measures exist cover many of the endpoints of CAM treatments. Existing measures can be and have been used in studies of the effectiveness of treatments involving CAM. Some subjective domains are more unique to specific CAM modalities (e.g., feelings of "centeredness" or "wholeness") and some additional measurement work may be required for these modalities; but in principle, virtually any subjective experience can be captured either as present or absent or as present as a matter of degree.

Because subjective experiences cannot be independently validated, and because they can be significantly affected by context, contrast, and expectation effects, it is particularly important to try to build in features of the study design that minimize these kinds of biases. "Blinding" the patient to the specific treatment that he or she has received, for example, is a way to minimize the effects of expectations on reports of subjective outcomes. Careful selection of patients who are all similar in terms of the level of pain or disability at the time of treatment is a way to minimize contrast effects. Having the outcome assessment done by a person other than the treating clinician is a way to minimize the biasing effects from the desire of a patient to please the clinician.

Objective Outcomes

Objective outcomes include those things that can be felt, seen, heard, or measured in some way by someone other than the patient. Status as alive or dead, weight, blood pressure, tumor size, white blood cell counts, and levels of blood sugar all represent examples of objective measures used regularly in treatment effectiveness studies. In conventional medicine, the vast range of tests possible in the domains of laboratory tests, radiologic and nuclear imaging, physical examination, electrical recording (electrocardiograms, electroencephalograms, and electromyograms) are all potential means of obtaining objective outcome measures for specific treatments.

Even though the data for objective outcomes can often be stored and made available for repeat testing by other observers (e.g., two independent radiologists reading the same X-ray image), there is still some potential for bias, particularly if the person providing a treatment or studying its effects is the person performing a test or interpreting the results of a test. Many objective tests still involve some judgment or interpretation on the part of the person performing or interpreting the test, so it is important to design effectiveness studies in ways that minimize any biasing effects of those judgments or interpretations. The most common way to minimize bias is to make sure that the person reading an X-ray image, taking and recording a blood pressure, or interpreting an electroencephalogramm is not someone with a vested interest in the results of a study and to try, whenever possible, to blind the person doing the test to any knowledge of the study treatment that the patient has received. Doing these two things minimizes the opportunity for any systematic bias either for or against a particular treatment being studied.

To the extent that treatments involving CAM are designed to influence objective endpoints like survival, blood pressure, tumor size, or the alignment and spacing of vertebrae, standard measures of these endpoints, with appropriate blinding and other controls for bias, should be suitable for treatment effectiveness research in CAM.

CONTEMPORARY ISSUES IN STUDY DESIGN AND ANALYSIS

In the last 10 to 15 years, a consensus has emerged about the types of scientific evidence required to establish the efficacy or the effectiveness of a treatment. Doctors and patients adopt health interventions, such as a CAM therapy, because someone will pay the cost (such as an insurance company or Medicare) and because the benefits of the intervention sufficiently outweigh its harms. These benefits and harms are the *outcomes* of the use of the intervention. The outcomes movement or the evidence-based medicine movement in health care is simply the application of the principle that societal and individual acceptance of a health care intervention should depend on the balance of its benefits, harms, and costs. The measurement of those benefits and harms, the balance of harms and benefits, and how that balance compares with the balance of harms and benefits of an established treatment are at the heart of most clinical research. This section discusses some core principles in comparisons and evaluations of health care interventions.

Many possible solutions or interventions exist for every human complaint and every affliction. Some interventions gain general acceptance and become standard treatment. Some of these have strong scientific evidence to support their use. That is, investigators have tested formal hypotheses about the interventions according to established principles and have found that they are clearly superior. Others have little or no scientific evidence to support their use but have become accepted as effective because of their long-term use. For practicing clinicians, clinical research often addresses the question asked by many patients, "This treatment has worked for me in the past, so why should I switch to another, less established treatment?" The way to answer this question is a head-to-head comparison of the two treatments. In designing a study to this end and analyzing the results, a number of considerations can be important. This section describes some of these considerations, with particular emphasis on how they apply to the problem of predicting the response to an intervention.

Predicting the Response to an Intervention

The data set from a randomized study of two treatments will contain many different variables. Among them is a measure of outcome (e.g., blood pressure at the end of the study); this variable would be the dependent variable in a multivariable model (the goal of the model would be to predict the end-of-study blood pressure). Another variable would be treatment assignment (Drug A or Drug B); treatment assignment would be a predictor variable (or an independent variable). Other predictor variables might include age, sex, ethnicity, pretreatment blood pressure, and dietary salt intake. One form of a multivariable model would include all of the predictor variables and might show that several predictor variables were significant predictors of the end-of-study blood pressure. One of them would be Drug A and another might be salt intake. In a multivariable regression model, these two would be independent predictors of outcome. This result would not prove that salt intake was a mediator of the response to Drug A, in the sense that Drug A had a greater effect in the presence of a low-salt diet versus high-salt diet. However, the model could be set up in a different way, with so-called interaction terms reflecting the extent to which the effects of Drug A and salt intake vary as the levels of the other variables vary. If the regression coefficient for this interaction term was significantly different from 0, a researcher could say that the interaction between Drug A and salt intake was a predictor of end-of-study blood pressure. In other words, the effect of Drug A on blood pressure was not the same for all levels of salt intake, and the effect of salt intake on blood pressure differed as a function of Drug A's presence or absence. The search for predictors of response would involve a search for significant interaction terms between the intervention and the predictor variables.

Stability of Predictive Models

A key element of a predictive model is its stability (its ability to give the same result if the study was repeated with a new sample of patients). One of the ways to predict the stability of a model is to count the number of outcome events. If the number of outcome events is small relative to the number of predictor variables in the model (a ratio of at least 10 outcome events per predictor variable is the minimum), the model is likely to be unstable. Thus, a model for the prediction of mortality after a surgical procedure would likely be unstable if the study recorded 15 deaths and the predictive model tested 8 variables. For this model to be stable, at least 80 deaths should have occurred. The reason that a model's stability depends on the ratio of the number of outcome events to the number of predictor variables is that small samples are likely to differ from the parent population to a greater degree than large samples would (the law of small numbers). One needs substantial numbers of people who experience the outcome, because statistical models for the identification of which potential predictors are good predictors rely upon differences in the frequencies of the potential predictors of outcome in those who experience the outcome and those who do not.

Distinguishing Between Intermediate and Distal Outcomes

It is important for researchers to decide whether to be satisfied with measuring intermediate outcomes (outcomes that predict death or long-term disability but that are not death or long-term disability themselves) as a result of an intervention or whether to measure the effects of the intervention on the death and disability rates of those diseases directly (distal outcomes). The treatment of hypertension is an informative example. One can compare two antihypertensive drugs by their effects on blood pressure; or one can compare their effects by determining the rates of strokes, congestive heart failure, or myocardial infarction between the two groups of patients taking the two drugs. Blood pressure is an intermediate outcome, of interest mostly because it predicts outcomes that frighten patients, such as stroke rates. It is much easier and much less costly to measure blood pressure than it is to measure stroke rates, which are typically small and which require many patient-years of monitoring for accurate measurement. Once several studies show, however, that lower blood pressure predicts fewer strokes, the decision to pay for a new antihypertensive drug might well rest on its effect on blood pressure, with the implicit assumption that the lower blood pressures brought about by treatment with the new drug relative to those achieved with standard therapy imply that the patients will experience fewer strokes. Therefore, although distal outcomes mean more to patients, it may not be necessary to measure them to determine whether a new drug is equal to or better than the standard therapy. The usefulness of intermediate outcomes in clinical research rests on the bedrock of a scientifically proven connection between the intermediate outcome and the distal outcome. It involves the assumption that the effect of a drug on blood pressure is the only determinant of stroke rates. A drug that affected blood pressure and blood clotting might have a greater effect on stroke rates than its effect on blood pressure would predict.

Standard Outcome Instruments Versus Customized Instruments

The rationale for standardizing measures of outcome rests upon the value placed on being able to compare the effects of different interventions. Compartmentalization of health care policy is shortsighted in the long run. For example, Medicare could be concerned about whether to pay for left ventricular assist devices for damaged hearts. If resources are limited, Medicare should consider alternative uses of the money expended on left ventricular devices. If decision makers ask, "What must we give up in order to pay for X?" they need a method that they can use to compare the interventions for one disease with the interventions for another disease.

The growth of standardized outcome measurements is a response to the need to compare the effects of treating diseases that have different outcomes. How does one compare a treatment for diabetes with a treatment for back pain? One uses some measure that both diseases affect, such as ability to function in daily life (the SF-36 questionnaire or activities of daily living). Instruments such as the SF-36 have been used in so many studies that scores serve as a way to compare one study population with another. Many disease-specific instruments are also available.

Cost-Effectiveness

Cost-effectiveness analysis is an important tool for evaluating health care interventions. According to Garber et al. (1997), cost-effectiveness is "a method designed to assess the comparative impact of expenditures on different health outcomes." The importance of cost-effectiveness is its salience to setting policies in a setting in which resources are constrained and people must make choices that involve trading off costs against effectiveness.

The salient word in describing cost-effectiveness analysis is "comparative." The cost-effectiveness of one intervention is always in relation to the cost-effectiveness of something else, even if the alternative is doing nothing. The cost-effectiveness of Intervention A compared with Intervention B is

$$\text{Cost-effectiveness} = (\text{cost}_A - \text{cost}_B)/(\text{QALY}_A - \text{QALY}_B)$$

where effectiveness is measured in clinical units and where QALY represents a quality-adjusted life year. A QALY is a year living in a specific state of health relative to the most desirable health state, usually perfect health. The relationship between a desirable health state and a less desirable one is a number, called a *utility*, which expresses the ratio of the patient's preference for a specific health state compared with that for perfect health. Thus, if the patient says a year with heart failure is equivalent to 80 percent of a year spent in perfect health, the utility for heart failure is 0.8. Thus, a year spent by one person living with heart failure counts as "0.8 QALY" and a year spent in perfect health counts as "1.0 QALY." In large populations of people, one can calculate the total number of QALYs that the population experiences over a period of time by adding the QALY values accumulated by each individual in the population over the time period being considered.

When one expresses effectiveness in QALYs, it is possible to compare several different interventions directly (e.g., the treatment of hypertension and screening for lung cancer). This advantage is very important for health care planning, in which those who provide or pay for health care assemble a package of health care interventions, because one can choose interventions on the basis of cost-effectiveness and obtain a package of services whose components have values—expressed as the health benefits obtained for the money expended—that are consistent with one another.

The analyst could express cost-effectiveness differently (e.g., the cost per patient death postponed or the cost per case of lung cancer detected). These methods are easier, but their use means that the power to compare interventions for two entirely different health conditions is given up. Estimation of the effect of an intervention on life expectancy, especially when life expectancy is adjusted for quality of life, requires a great deal more work, but most cost-effectiveness analyses calculate the cost per QALY.

In a typical cost-effectiveness analysis, the analyst uses a mathematical model to represent the alternative actions (e.g., a treatment, a clinical test, or observation) and their health consequences. The analyst represents the uncertainty of future events (e.g., death or survival after surgery) as a probability ranging from 0 to 1, and the outcome of various sets of events as a health state (e.g., death or survival with heart failure). The value of a given health state at a point in time is expressed on a 0-1 scale as a "utility," and the cumulative values of health states over a fixed period of time are expressed as quality-adjusted life years (QALY) (time spent in a given health state times the value placed on life in the health state).

Measurement of Preferences

The QALY is a key element of cost-effectiveness analysis because it expresses length of life in a common unit: healthy years. By using a common unit, one can compare the desirabilities of two different health states. To compare two outcome states quantitatively, one must characterize each one by a number that reflects the desirability of the outcome state. This number is the utility of the health state, usually expressed on a scale from 0 to 1. Several methods that can be used to elicit a person's utility for a health state exist. In many cost-effectiveness analyses, the researchers adopt a utility obtained from large population-based surveys (Torrance, 1986, 1987). The first method, the standard reference gamble method, is the most theoretically sound method but is also the most difficult for a patient to do. The second method, the time trade-off method, in which the patient is asked how many years in a particular health state are equivalent to the patient's life expectancy in perfect health is easier. With this method a patient is asked, "How many of your 20 years of expected life in your current health state would you give up to have perfect health for the rest of your life?" The third method is the easiest but is the least sound theoretically: "Point to a place on a scale from 0 to 10 that characterizes your feeling about a health state."

Do Outcomes Differ? Statistical Analysis

Study populations are necessarily samples of the universe of people who are eligible for a study. If the study population is small, the outcomes are more likely to differ by chance from the outcomes that would occur in the universe from which the sample was drawn. Because the results from any one sample can be atypical, scientists use the concept of the 95 percent confidence interval, which is the range of outcomes that would occur in 95 of 100 samples from the universe. One can calculate the 95 percent confidence interval for the difference between two outcomes. If the 95 percent confidence interval for the difference includes 0 (no difference), the results of the study that gave rise to the difference are consistent with no difference. Statistical tests estimate the probability that a difference in outcomes is consistent with chance, usually expressed as the "*p* value." Outcome studies increasingly report the confidence interval of the absolute difference in outcomes related to two interventions. This method provides a graphic measure of the uncertainty in a conclusion. If the confidence interval of the difference includes 0 or a value that is very close to 0, the difference is not statistically significant or is of borderline statistical significance, respectively. If the lower limit of the confidence interval of the difference is far from 0, one can be sure that the difference itself is unlikely to be the product of a chance variation in the samples drawn from the same universe.

Confidence intervals enter into the interpretation of predictive models designed to identify clinical predictors of a response to a treatment, such as an element of a package of CAM interventions for a clinical problem. The coefficient of an interaction term has a confidence interval. If it includes 0, the interaction term is not a statistically significant predictor of the dependent variable (e.g., Drug A, salt intake, and end-of-study blood pressure, as in the earlier example).

Measurement Error

Measurement error adds uncertainty. The inclusion of a measurement error widens the 95 percent confidence interval. Failure to take into account measurement error will lead one to overestimate precision and draw incorrect conclusions about differences in outcomes.

Effectiveness Versus Efficacy Studies

Efficacy Studies

Efficacy studies mean, by common agreement, that the comparison of two technologies has taken place under strictly controlled conditions designed to show a difference if a difference is truly present. Typically, an efficacy study will exclude patients who are likely to die of diseases other than the target disease for the technology under study to maximize the information value of each death in characterizing the two technologies. The study population of an efficacy study is typically narrowly defined (and therefore relatively small), which means that the patients are very similar to one another and, therefore, that the results may not apply to a wider population. All measurements take place under optimum conditions, and the doctors interpreting the test results undergo special training so that they give the same interpretation, for example, to the same computed tomography scan, eliminating one source of measurement error. Typically, efficacy studies precede effectiveness studies, and the results are used as a "proof of principle." After proof of principle, other studies may explore the size of the effect in different study populations, at different clinical sites, and under different conditions of practice. These are effectiveness studies.

Effectiveness Studies

Effectiveness studies evaluate the technology under real-world conditions of actual medical practice. The study population resembles that which one would see in day-to-day clinical practice, which means that any results are likely to apply to real-world clinical practice. Effectiveness studies have a greater chance of measurement error if the researchers have taken few precautions to standardize the measurements. Although measurement error reduces the precision of effectiveness studies, study populations are typically large, which increases the statistical precision.

Noninferiority and Superiority Trials

Some researchers want to prove that their product is better than the standard product. If the new product is very effective, relatively small study populations may suffice to prove that the product is superior to the standard product. Often, however, researchers are content to show that their product is equivalent to the standard product. A typical situation is a minor chemical variation to a standard drug. The minor variation means that the patent on the standard drug does not apply, and the company making the new product can market it, as long as it is as good as the standard product. Thus, some studies are designed to prove noninferiority (the product is highly likely to be as good as the standard product). The designer of the trial tries to estimate the number of patients required to show that the two products do not result in clinically important differences in outcomes. One means to this end is to include enough subjects to be sure that the upper limit of the 95 percent confidence interval of the difference in outcomes (the largest difference that is reasonably possible) is slightly smaller than the minimum clinically important difference in outcomes. This technique almost guarantees that if the two products are truly equivalent, any difference actually observed between them in a particular study will be less than the smallest difference that clinicians would find meaningful. For all intents, the two interventions have equivalent effects.

Co-Morbidity and Cointerventions as Confounders

Suppose one is investigating the relationship between eating a particular brand of breakfast cereal and subsequent myocardial infarction. The greater the intake of the cereal is, the greater the incidence of myocardial infarction is. Is eating the cereal associated with myocardial infarction? Now, suppose that cereal eaters and noneaters also differ in the prevalence of diabetes, with more cases of diabetes occurring in the cereal-eating population. The presence of diabetes is confounding the relationship between cereal eating and myocardial infarction. Diabetes is thus a *"co-morbid condition,"* a form of confounder.

Medications can also confound a relationship. Suppose that one studies the effects of two blood pressure medications on heart failure. Since high blood pressure is a cause of heart failure, the study will be stronger if the blood pressure in the two study groups is the same. So, the researchers allow the doctors caring for the patients to use medications in addition to the study medications to get a patient's blood pressure to a target level. The other blood pressure medications are *"cointerventions."* Cointerventions can be confounders if they affect the outcome state, which is heart failure in this example. If the researchers do not adjust for differences in the cointervention medications, which may vary throughout the study, they may form an incorrect conclusion about the relationship of the study medication to heart failure. That is, what appears to be an effect of the study medication may be an effect of the cointervention.

Single-Center Versus Multicenter Studies

Studies that take place in many different clinical sites are increasingly the norm for the testing of major hypotheses about treatments for disease. One reason is sample size. More sites mean more patients, which means greater statistical precision and the ability to make strong statistical inferences about relatively small (and even clinically unimportant) differences (of course, one may lose statistical precision if the clustering of outcomes occurs, but a good study design will allow a larger sample size so that clustering does not reduce the statistical power of a study). The use of more study sites means greater variability in the patients and in clinical care and less risk that the differences between two interventions are due to idiosyncrasies of practice at a single site rather than the intervention itself. The use of more study sites also means that more investigators are talking among themselves and finding ways to strengthen the study that a single investigator might miss. A study at more sites also means greater costs, which often make a study infeasible without a corporate sponsor. Alternatively, the greater costs may mean less thorough data collection and a greater risk that the findings from the study will not be interpretable at its conclusion. Despite the costs, multicenter studies are the norm for the testing of important hypotheses. Relatively few studies of CAM interventions have been performed at multiple sites, so this form of research is an untapped opportunity for CAM researchers.

Clustering of Outcomes

Conventional statistical methods assume that the outcomes for individual patients are independent of one another, so that each patient contributes new additional information about the relationship of an outcome to the two interventions. When the care given by different providers (either institutions or doctors) results in different outcomes, outcomes are said to be "clustered." When a study takes place in several different institutions, which is common practice, it is possible that care provided at each of the institutions differs, so that knowledge of what institution is providing the care allows one to predict the outcomes for the patients. Under these circumstances, the outcome for each study patient is not independent of those for other patients at that institution, and the assumptions of conventional statistical methods do not hold. The assumption of independence when outcomes are related means that measures of variability, such as the 95 percent confidence interval, appear to be more precise than they really are. The true 95 percent confidence interval is wider than it appears to be from the findings of the study, which means that an apparent true difference may be consistent with random variation between the study patients who receive the intervention and those who do not. The use of an appropriate statistical design can account for the effects of clustering, so that the statistical power of the study and the widths of resulting confidence intervals are accurately known. Widening of the 95 percent confidence interval after this statistical adjustment is made means that clustering of outcomes is present. Clustering of outcomes makes it more difficult to conclude that a difference between two interventions is due to the interventions rather than to chance variation.

Clustering of outcomes is especially important in studies in which the deployment of an intervention may vary from practitioner to practitioner or from study site to study site. CAM experts commonly cite the special role of the practitioner as a characteristic of CAM interventions, so it is important to know when outcomes vary in this way. If adjustment for clustering widens the confidence interval, the clustering of outcomes by provider or by site may be occurring. If some providers or sites are doing better (or worse), researchers have an opportunity to discover what makes certain providers or sites more effective.

LEVELS OF EVIDENCE

Hierarchies of Evidence

The U.S. Preventive Services Task Force (1996) and groups organized to develop treatment guidelines have adopted a concept of "levels of evidence" or a "hierarchy of evidence" that they use to rate the strength of the

TABLE 3-1 The Evidence Rating System of the U.S. Preventive Services Task Force

---

Overall rating
- Good
- Fair
- Poor

Definition of "good"
- Consistent results
- Well designed, well conducted
- Representative populations
- Directly assesses effects on health outcomes

Definition of "fair"
- Evidence adequate to determine effects on health outcomes but limited by
  —Number, quality, or consistency of studies
  —Generalizability to routine practice
  —Indirect character of the effect on health outcomes

Definition of "poor"
- Evidence is *insufficient* to assess effects on health outcomes because
  —Limited number of studies
  —Limited power of studies (a wide 95 percent confidence interval that leads to inconclusive results)
  —Important flaws in study design or conduct
  —Gaps in the chain of evidence
  —Lack of information on health outcomes

---

body of published data on a specific test or treatment. The Task Force's approach to rating evidence appears in Table 3-1. Note that it does not use a hierarchy of study designs ranging from the most powerful (randomized clinical trials) to the weakest (case series). Rather, it uses generic characteristics of a study and of a group of studies. In effect, the term "well designed" reflects a hierarchy of study designs, but a hierarchy is not an explicit part of the Task Force's evidence hierarchy.

The principal product of the U.S. Preventive Services Task Force is recommendations for using preventive interventions in office-based clinical practice. The Task Force has a hierarchy of rating of the strengths of recommendations, which it has refined over the two decades of its existence. The hierarchy of the strengths of recommendations is important because practitioners, health care organizations, and payers pay attention to the Task Force's recommendations. An explicit hierarchy of recommendations with definitions that are tied to the strength of evidence makes the Task Force accountable for the strength of its recommendations. A system of accountability reduces the chance that the Task Force will make an arbitrary recommendation. The hierarchy of strengths of recommendations appears in Table 3-2.

TABLE 3-2 Strength of Recommendation and Strength of Evidence, U.S. Preventive Services Task Force

---

A Strongly recommend
  • *Good* evidence; benefits substantially outweigh harms
B Recommend
  • At least *fair* evidence; benefits outweigh harms
C U.S. Preventive Services Task Force makes no recommendation
  • *Fair to good* evidence; benefits and harms closely balanced
D Recommend against routine use
  • Ineffective or harms outweigh potential benefits
E Insufficient evidence to recommend for or against
  • Lack of evidence on clinical outcomes
  • *Poor* quality of existing studies
  • *Good* quality studies with conflicting results
  • Confidence interval includes clinically important benefits

---

Another hierarchy of evidence, from the National Health Service Centre for Evidence-Based Medicine, appears in Table 3-3. In contrast to the U.S. Preventive Services Task Force hierarchy, this hierarchy depends on the study design, the number of studies in the body of evidence, and the consistency of study results. In this hierarchy, the combined results of several randomized controlled clinical trials (RCTs) receive the greatest weight in evaluating treatment effectiveness. The results of a single, well-designed RCT is given the next greatest weight. The combined results of observational studies or other non-RCT study designs comes next, followed by case series or anecdotal reports, and professional judgment or consensus.

A recent IOM report (2001) proposed a slightly different approach to levels of evidence for research when the question considered is one of treatment effectiveness rather than efficacy. First, that report describes using an "effectiveness RCT." Such a study would have the following characteristics:

• light patient exclusion criteria;
• conducted in a range of treatment settings;
• treatment provided by the kinds of providers who would provide treatment in non-study settings;
• no elaborate data collection (e.g., extra lab test or imaging studies);
• analysis done on "intention to treat" basis; and
• random assignment with one or more control groups.

Further, that report takes the position that when evaluating treatment effectiveness, "the results of a single well-designed outcomes study should

TABLE 3-3 Example of a Hierarchy of Evidence from the National Health Service Centre for Evidence-Based Medicine, 2002

An A-level recommendation for therapy
- Level 1a evidence
  —Systematic review of many RCTs (with homogeneity)
- Level 1b evidence
  —A single RCT with narrow confidence intervals
- Level 1c evidence
  —Case series of a disease from which all patients died before the new treatment; now some survive
  —Case series of a disease from which many patients died before the new treatment; now all survive

A B-level recommendation for therapy
- Level 2a evidence
  —Systematic review of many cohort studies (with homogeneity)
- Level 2b evidence
  —A single-cohort study
  - Includes randomized clinical trial with >20 percent drop-outs
- Level 2c evidence
  —Ecological studies (performed with a preexisting dataset)

- Level 3a evidence
  —Systematic review of many case-control studies (with homogeneity)
- Level 3b evidence
  —A single case-control study

A C-level recommendation for therapy
- Level 4 evidence
  —Case series
  —Poor-quality cohort and case-control studies

A D-level recommendation for therapy
- Level 5 evidence
  —Expert opinion without an explicit critical appraisal of the evidence
  —Expert opinion based on
  - Physiology
  - Bench research
  - "First principles"

SOURCE: Adapted from Phillips et al. (1999).

be considered to be as compelling as the results of a single well-controlled randomized trial" (IOM, 2001) and lays out a hierarchy of evidence as shown in Table 3-4.

In this report about CAM, the committee has chosen not to recommend one particular hierarchy; however, it does emphasize the following points:

TABLE 3-4 Hierarchy of Evidence

Level	Emphasis on Efficacy	Emphasis on Effectiveness
I	Systematic Review (e.g., meta-analysis of Several Well-Controlled Randomized Trials—consistent results	Systematic Review (e.g., meta-analysis) of Several Well-Designed Outcome Studies or "Effectiveness RCTs"—consistent results
II	Single Well-Controlled Randomized Trial	Single Well-Designed Outcomes Study or "Effectiveness RCT"
III	Consistent Findings from Multiple Cohort, Case-Control, or Observational Studies	
IV	Single Cohort, Case-Control, or Observational Study	
V	Uncontrolled Experiment, Unsystematic Observation, Expert Opinion, or Consensus Judgments	

SOURCE: IOM, 2001.

- In general an RCT is the preferred study design if the issue is establishing treatment efficacy.
- More studies are better than fewer studies, therefore a meta-analysis of multiple good RCTs is better than one good RCT.
- Other study designs can provide evidence of efficacy or effectiveness.
- Meta-analysis of multiple non-RCT studies is better than one non-RCT study. Meta-analysis of multiple non-RCT studies may or may not be better than one good RCT; it depends on the details of the studies and the specific question being asked.
- If the question is treatment effectiveness, then some features of the typical RCT (stringent inclusion/exclusion criteria; treatment given in high-quality, high-volume clinical sites; detailed, frequent patient follow-up; etc.) create problems in generalizing findings to routine practice settings.
- Other study designs, including observational studies or "effectiveness RCTs," may provide evidence that is at least equally compelling as that provided by an "efficacy RCT."

Effect size is another consideration that must be taken into account along with features of study design when one weighs the strength of evidence for a particular therapy. Treatments with clear, dramatic, positive effects in small or less well-controlled studies may be deemed "efficacious" sooner than treatments with more modest effects.

APPLYING CONTEMPORARY RESEARCH METHODS TO CAM

The remainder of this chapter discusses the context in which researchers will apply these established research methods, including the idea that CAM users may present particular needs for research, that CAM interventions may pose particular problems in applying research methods that have worked well for conventional medicine, and that such interventions may also expose some of the weaknesses of applying contemporary research practices to conventional medicine.

Decision Makers and Sources of Evidence

Lewith and colleagues (2001) have described the different decisions that various participants in health care make about treatments and how they use different kinds of information to make those decisions. Patients, providers, insurers, government policy makers, and others typically require different types of evidence and different amounts of certainty to decide for or against a particular treatment or treatment modality. The committee recognized that a discussion of evidence of CAM treatment effectiveness must be set in the context of the differences among users of information about CAM in terms of the decisions that they make, the information that they need to make those decisions, and the way(s) in which they think about treatment effectiveness.

Researchers

Researchers are typically interested in understanding cause-and-effect relationships between underlying mechanisms of illness, treatments designed to alter those mechanisms, and patient outcomes. Researchers trained in Western cultures and scientific traditions generally think in terms of linear cause-and-effect and try to identify the simplest possible causal models (i.e., the fewest explanatory variables and the simplest relationships among those variables) that account for the observed associations (Nisbett, 2003). Scientists from other cultures, however, may be more likely to think in terms of more complex "system" models that involve multiple factors and multiple levels of relationships and highly interactive and iterative, rather than linear, relationships (Nisbett, 2003).

The results of a given study are taken as evidence of cause-and-effect relationships to the extent that certain criteria are met. These criteria typically include

• Features of the study design that allow strong inferences to be made about cause-and-effect relationships:

— a well-defined population to whom the conclusions apply;

— a well-defined, sufficiently large, and representative sample drawn from that population;

— a well-defined and controlled treatment(s) administration;

— a concurrent control or comparison group(s), when possible, that receives either no treatment or some different form or dose of the study treatment;

— well-defined study endpoints (objectively defined and measured outcome variables); and

— statistical analysis to assess the likelihood that the findings are produced by chance.

• Plausible biological mechanisms, that is, the ability to fit the observed relationships into some larger body of theory and evidence on how the body works.

• Consistency of findings from study to study. A single study is rarely definitive, although some large, well-designed clinical trials may produce evidence that is treated by the scientific community as definitive. Confidence in the existence of cause-and-effect relationships grows with the ability to see them in multiple studies over time. Confidence diminishes when results vary from study to study.

• Dose-response relationships. In most biological processes, the introduction of a larger amount of a substance produces a larger subsequent effect. There is almost always some upper limit at which no further effect is found or some different or counterbalancing biological process begins to take over. For the most part, however, within a reasonable range of doses, more "cause" produces more "effect." Clear dose-response relationships typically increase the confidence in the underlying causal relationships between the treatment and the outcome.

Teachers Training New Practitioners

Medical school, nursing school, and allied health school faculty require evidence of treatment effectiveness to determine how to train students. The standards of evidence for specific treatments are not necessarily the same as those used by researchers, but they are similar. They include

• The criteria for researchers listed above. Faculty have the responsibility to stay current with the published literature and generally to apply the same criteria to published studies that researchers apply.

• Personal experience. In addition, however, clinical faculty draw heavily on their own experiences in determining which treatments are effective and which ones are not. This may be particularly true in the context of clinical rotations and residency training, in which much teaching is done on the basis of an apprenticeship model in a specific clinical environment. In this setting, both faculty and students have a chance to observe, directly and together, the effectiveness of specific treatments.

• The extent to which the treatment in question is a "standard of practice" in the medical community or is moving toward that standing. Students entering a profession become part of a professional community, and part of their learning involves knowing what the standards and typical practices of that community are. There is often a gap in time between the publication of scientific evidence of the effectiveness of a new treatment and the widespread adoption of that treatment by most or all members of a professional community, along with some appropriate caution and skepticism about new findings that seem to run counter to daily experience. Teachers train students in what the members of the professional community typically *do* on a daily basis as well as what the published literature says that they *could* or *should* do.

Practicing Clinicians

Clinicians treating patients have a somewhat more complex set of information requirements about treatment effectiveness, because they must know not only what has worked or what should have been effective in the abstract but also what they are actually able to do in the context of their own training and skills, their own practice settings, and their own sets of patients. Their requirements for information on treatment effectiveness include

• All of the preceding criteria, although many active clinicians will not have the same amount of time as their researcher or faculty colleagues do to monitor developments in the published literature.

• Consistency of a new practice with other aspects of current practice. A psychotherapist may accept the published evidence about the effectiveness of a specific herb for the treatment of depression but may be unwilling to incorporate the use of the herb into his or her own practice because of a professional commitment to therapies based on a different theory and conceptual model of mental illness.

• The availability of essential equipment, trained staff, supplies, and anything else necessary to provide a treatment safely and effectively. Many treatments require specialized equipment, training, or support staff that are not readily available to all clinicians.

• Difficulty in learning new skills (e.g., for new surgical procedures).

• The acceptability of a new treatment to patients and others in the community. Health care is usually a two-way human interaction; and potentially effective treatments will not be used if they conflict with the beliefs, cultural values, or expectations of large numbers of patients in a practice.

• Opinions of professional peers. In an environment in which it is impossible to keep up with all new advances in treatment, the opinions and practices of respected colleagues are a kind of evidence of treatment effectiveness that is often dominant.

• Reimbursement policies affecting a new treatment. Even when all other criteria have been met, a new treatment may not be adopted if the provision of it will not be adequately reimbursed.

• The extent to which the patient population is similar to those studied in clinical trials or other studies of treatment effectiveness. There are always variations in published studies of treatment effectiveness, and clinicians may legitimately believe that what works for many or most patients will not necessarily work for their own patients, particularly if they share some clinically relevant characteristic (Park, 2002).

Employers or Purchasers and Insurers

Those who pay for health care through insurance care about effectiveness, but also about cost-effectiveness, since they have at least some responsibility to use the dollars available for insurance to produce the best possible health benefit for covered employees. Evidence of treatment effectiveness relevant to employers and insurers, then, includes

• The scientific evidence listed above for researchers.

• The preferences, expectations, and experiences of employees and their families. Employers are not insuring passive and uninformed people. Employees who have positive experiences with specific therapies will ask for such therapies to be covered by insurance plans and may use coverage for those therapies as the basis for choosing one plan over another at open enrollment or even changing jobs.

• Published cost-effectiveness studies (when available). Employers and insurers may legitimately refuse to cover treatments that are effective but that are so costly that their inclusion prevents the coverage of less costly treatments that provide more health benefit to larger numbers of people.

• Internal cost-effectiveness analyses (for some larger employers). Large companies with many thousands of employees may be able to use their own databases to study relationships between treatments and work attendance, productivity, or the costs of illness. This information may be more compelling than information in published studies because there is no question about the generalizability of the findings to that employer's population.

Patients and Consumers

Individual patients generally do not have direct access to peer-reviewed journals, and most patients do not have the technical background to interpret the results of published treatment-effectiveness studies. This information tends to be filtered through someone else before it reaches the individual patient. In addition, patients (particularly those with chronic conditions) have their own experiences to draw on and can judge treatment effectiveness by the extent to which their own symptoms or functional status improve with treatment. Information on treatment effectiveness for individual patients, then, comes mainly from

- Information provided by a clinician(s) in one-on-one treatment encounters,
- Word of mouth from friends and relatives,
- The lay press or media,
- Direct-to-consumer advertising,
- Internet,
- Direct personal experience (particularly for patients with chronic conditions), and
- Communications from illness advocacy groups.

The Application of Contemporary Clinical Research Methods to CAM: Some Cautions

Although the concept of levels of evidence has generally been accepted and widely used in many domains of conventional medicine, some question its applicability to CAM therapies or to individual treatment decisions for specific patients. These questions particularly relate to the use of RCTs as the "gold standard" of evidence. Given the broad array of modalities that are included within the definition of CAM, it may be that some CAM therapies are more amenable to evaluation than others. Questions about the applicability of clinical research methods to CAM are described and discussed below.

Emphasis on Efficacy Rather Than Effectiveness

As noted above, the distinction between efficacy and effectiveness refers to the extent to which a treatment has a measurable positive effect in highly controlled clinical trial contexts (efficacy) versus whether the treatment has a measurable positive effect in routine daily clinical practice with unselected clinicians and patients (effectiveness). Efficacy refers to what a treatment *can* do under ideal circumstances; effectiveness refers to what a treatment *does* do in routine daily use. Because the highest level of evidence in most evidence hierarchies is the combined results of several RCTs, the resulting recommendations will inevitably be based on evidence of efficacy rather than evidence of effectiveness.

Difficult to Apply to Therapies for Which RCTs Are Difficult, Expensive, or Unethical

It may be impossible to organize RCTs in situations in which the effects to be observed occur rarely, take many years to develop, or are relatively subtle. It is also difficult to conduct RCTs in situations in which the treatment is already in wide use and is generally accepted as effective. It may also be difficult or impossible to randomize patients to CAM modalities or specific therapies that inherently depend on patients' belief, faith, or confidence in or relationship with a particular modality or provider. (See the discussion of "preference trials" in Chapter 4 for one way to address this problem.)

Hard to Apply to Treatments That Become Popular and Widely Used Very Quickly

Study participants may not accept random assignment to a placebo or some other type of control groups if the general public believes that the treatment being studied is widely effective. Likewise, institutional review boards may not be willing to approve randomization to a placebo or another control group if the professional community believes that the therapy being studied is widely effective. In addition to the problem of organizing RCTs for widely used treatments, there may also be a problem with all other study designs that involve some form of control condition that involves administration of a possibly ineffective treatment.

Relatively Long Delay from First Development of a Treatment to Assembly of Large Body of Evidence

The FDA has requirements for research on new drugs before they can be prescribed, but there are no similar requirements for surgical procedures and most CAM modalities. In both cases, there may be a long time lag (several years, in some instances) between the development and the first use of a treatment and the assembly of a body of scientific evidence of effectiveness. For drugs, this lag is invisible to most of the general public, and some evidence from RCTs must have been assembled before a drug is allowed on the market. For other treatments, however, the time required to organize an RCT or collect the results of other types of studies means that a large body of anecdotal experience will have been developed before more formal scientific evidence appears. For many CAM therapies based on traditional cultural beliefs, this time lag may be measured in hundreds of years.

Emphasis on What's Best for Largest Number Rather Than Search for What's Best for Unique, Individual Patients

A treatment is judged effective in an RCT if it is better than a placebo or an alternative form of treatment. "Better" means that the average outcome for the experimental group is superior to that for a control group, as determined by statistical tests that relate the difference in average outcomes to the variation in outcomes in the two groups. Unless the differences between the experimental group and the control group are dramatic, however, there are usually some patients in the experimental group who do worse than some patients in the control group (Park, 2002). What is best, then, for the "typical" or "average" patient is not necessarily best for *every* patient. This approach to identifying effective treatments is fundamentally different from the approach that emphasizes individual tailoring of treatments found in CAM modalities like homeopathy or traditional Chinese medicine.

The desire to have objective, well-defined study endpoints in RCTs can lead to a focus on health outcomes like mortality, tumor shrinkage, or change in a measurable physiological parameter like temperature or blood pressure. An exclusive focus on objective endpoints can lead researchers to miss or ignore other effects in the realm of subjective symptoms (e.g., pain, fatigue, and cognitive function) and general well-being. For many CAM therapies, the treatment goals include feelings of well-being and mastery of the illness (Jonas and Linde, 2002); these will not be captured in studies with more objectively defined primary endpoints.

Wellness Versus Treatment Effectiveness as a Research Objective

Recent national surveys (see Chapter 2; Astin, 1998; Astin et al., 2000) have highlighted the fact that many CAM "treatments" are not used to treat a specific current problem or disease but, rather, are used to either prevent disease or to promote a more general state of health and well-being. RCTs may still be used to assess the effects of CAM on general health or well-being, but such RCTs may be even more difficult to conduct than RCTs of the effectiveness of treatments for specific diseases. RCTs in the domain of disease prevention or wellness enhancement may require much longer time lines (e.g., 10 to 20 years or more), very large sample sizes because of the relatively low incidence of specific medical problems being prevented, or even larger sample sizes because of the potential of loss to follow-up or switching of treatment arms over the course of the study (i.e., patients randomized to the presumed active treatment quit taking or doing it, and patients randomized to the control arm begin to take or do the active treatment on their own). Some outcome variables may be hard to define and measure (e.g., "I just feel better"), and effect sizes may be small, again adding to the sample size required for a trial to have a reasonable chance of detecting an effect if it is truly present. Finally, patients will inevitably be doing several things that contribute to wellness (or lack of it) over a multiyear study period, and it will be difficult to isolate the effects of a CAM therapy or modality from the effects of a larger package of lifestyle factors.

REFERENCES

Astin JA. 1998. Why patients use alternative medicine: Results of a national study. *JAMA* 279(19):1548–1553.

Astin JA, Pelletier KR, Marie A, Haskell WL. 2000. Complementary and alternative medicine use among elderly persons: One-year analysis of a Blue Shield Medicare supplement. *J Gerontol A Biol Sci Med Sci* 55(1): M4–M9.

Bensen K and Hartz AJ. 2000. A comparison of observatonal studies and randomized controlled trials. *NEJM* 342(25):1878–1886.

Bowling A. 1997. *Measuring Health: A Review of Quality of Life Measurement Scales*. Philadelphia, PA: Open University Press.

Byar DP. 1980. Why data bases should not replace randomized clinical trials. *Biometrics*, (June), 36:337–342.

Cochrane AL. 1972. *Effectiveness and Efficiency: Random Reflections on Health Services*. London: Nuffield Provincial Hospitals Trust.

Farquhar C, Basser R, Hetrick S, Lethaby A, Marjoribanks J. 2003. High dose chemotherapy and autologous bone marrow or stem cell transplantation versus conventional chemotherapy for women with metastatic breast cancer. *Cochrane Database Syst Rev* (1):CD003142.

Frank-Stromborg M, Olsen SJ. 1997. *Instruments for Clinical Health Care Research*. Sudbury, MA: Jones and Bartlett.

Garber AM, Phelps CE. 1997. Economic foundations of cost-effectiveness analysis. *J Health Econ* 16:1–31.

IOM (Institute of Medicine). 2001. *Gulf War Veterans: Treating Symptoms and Syndromes*. Washington, DC: National Academy Press.

Jonas WB, Linde K. 2002. Conducting and Evaluating Clinical Research on Complementary and Alternative Medicine. In: Gallin JI, ed. *Principles and Practice of Clinical Research*. San Diego, CA: Academic Press. Pp. 401–426.

Kaptchuk TJ, Kerr CE. 2004. Commentary: Unbiased divination, unbiased evidence, and the patulin clinical trial. *Int J Epidemiol* 33(2):247–251.

Lewith GT, Hyland M, Gray SF. 2001. Attitudes to and use of complementary medicine among physicians in the United Kingdom. *Complement Ther Med* 9(3):167–172.

McDowell I, Newell C. 1996. *Measuring Health: A Guide to Rating Scales and Questionnaires*. New York: Oxford University Press.

McPherson K, Wennberg JE, Hovind OB, Clifford P. 1982. Small-area variations in the use of common surgical procedures: An international comparison of New England, England, and Norway. *N Engl J Med* 307(21):1310–1314.

Moseley JB, O'Malley K, Petersen NJ, Menke TJ, Brody BA, Kuykendall DH, Hollingsworth JC, Ashton CM, Wray NP. 2002. A controlled trial of arthroscopic surgery for osteoarthritis of the knee. *N Engl J Med* 347(2):81–88.

Neuhauser D. 2002. Heroes and martyrs of quality and safety: Ernest Armory Codman, MD. *Qual Saf Health Care* 11:104–105.

Nisbett RE. 2003. *The Geography of Thought: How Asians and Westerners Think Differently and Why*. New York: Free Press.

Park CM. 2002. Diversity, the individual, and proof of efficacy: Complementary and alternative medicine in medical education. *Am J Public Health* 92(10):1568–1572.

Phillips R, Ball C, Sackett D, Badenoch D, Straus S, Haynes B, Dawes M, McAlister FA. 2004. [Online]. Available: http://www.cebm.net/downloads/Oxford_CEBM_Levels_5.rtf [accessed May 2004].

Rossouw JE, Anderson GL, Prentice RL, LaCrois AZ, Kooperberg C, Stefanick ML, Jackson RD, Beresford SA, Howard BV, Johnson KC, Kotchen JM, Ockene J. 2002. Risks and benefits of estrogen plus progestin in healthy postmenopausal women: Principal results from the Women's Health Initiative randomized controlled trial. *JAMA* 288(3):321–333.

Torrance GW. 1986. Measurement of health state utilities for economic appraisal: A review. *J Health Econ* 5(1):1–30.

Upjohn Co. v. Finch. 422 F.2d 944, 955 (6th Cir. 1970).

U.S. Preventive Services Task Force. 1996. *Guide to Clinical Preventive Services*. Baltimore, MD: Williams & Wilkins.

U.S. Statutes at Large 65 (1951):648.

U.S. Statutes at Large 65 (1962):788–789.

Wennberg J, Gittelsohn A. 1982. Variations in medical care among small areas. *Sci Am* 246(4):120–134.

4

Need for Innovative Designs in Research on CAM and Conventional Medicine

CHARACTERISTICS OF CAM TREATMENTS AND MODALITIES

Standard randomized controlled trials (RCTs); which consist of two or three study arms, large numbers of patients in each study arm, one specific, standard treatment or dose of treatment per study arm, and 1 or 2 years of follow-up may be ill-suited to answer questions about the long-term effects of complementary and alternative medicine (CAM) therapies on disease prevention and wellness. Several characteristics of CAM treatments and modalities are also difficult to incorporate into treatment effectiveness studies with shorter time lines as well as studies with more clearly defined symptom relief or disease state endpoints. These characteristics are not unique to CAM and are further discussed below.

CAM modalities frequently use "bundles" of therapies rather than just one therapy in isolation. Survey data show that patients who use one CAM modality frequently use other CAM modalities at the same time and use CAM modalities along with conventional medicine treatments for the same condition (Eisenberg et al., 1993, 1998; Wolsko et al., 2002). Although it may be possible to enroll patients in a study that restricts their treatments to one at a time, it is difficult, scientifically questionable, and possibly even unethical to restrict for study purposes treatments that would naturally accompany the specific therapy or modality being studied. For example, it may be difficult to conduct an RCT of a specific massage therapy technique if a large fraction of patients who receive this treatment in routine practice would also receive various combinations of herbal therapies, aromatherapy, stretching and exercise recommendations, and relaxation therapies.

It is often difficult to define the thing to be studied. Patients receiving homeopathy might also be accurately described as receiving a particular type, class, or school of homeopathic treatment; treatment from a particular type of provider or individual provider; and treatment with a particular material or combination of materials. Research could conceivably be done to establish the effectiveness of any of these things, from the most general to the most specific. The level of analysis that would be most informative for clinicians, individual patients, or health policy makers is not obvious. This problem is occasionally encountered in conventional medicine but less commonly than in CAM, as questions about effectiveness typically pertain to very precisely defined therapies rather than to whole disciplines or schools of thought (e.g., medicine, surgery, or radiation therapy). As a matter of convenience, one may speak of a study comparing surgical and medical treatments for low back pain, but a study would typically define the treatments in each domain quite specifically and not presume to be evaluating all possible treatments that might be offered under those broad labels. In CAM, however, there is a greater tendency to pose research questions about the effectiveness of whole modalities or schools of thought; for example, does chiropractic work for back or neck pain, and does acupuncture work for headache?

In CAM, treatments are individualized for each patient, and treatments may be individualized for each patient at each treatment (Park, 2002) One reason that research questions may be posed about whole CAM modalities at a time is that in some CAM modalities (e.g., traditional Chinese medicine) there is no such thing as a "standard" treatment or dose. Individualization of therapy to a unique combination of patient characteristics is a core concept of the modality. The only common characterstics to be studied across multiple patients and generalized from a study sample to a larger universe of patients are the modality and the general approach taken by the practitioner. Everything else can and will vary from patient to patient, at least in principle.

Some treatments are presumed to depend on the unique characteristics of the healer and on features of the healer-patient relationship. In some of the energy or touch therapies, for example, qi gong, the effectiveness of the treatment is presumed to be inherently bound up in a skill or an ability of the healer that may be viewed as a gift and therefore not easily measurable or generalizable (Krieger, 1998). This is not a completely foreign concept to research in conventional medicine; studies of surgical procedures typically take the skill or experience of the surgeon into account in some way; and studies of psychotherapy may take into account some measure of the skill, empathy level, or experience of the therapist. It is a complicating factor for research in any study in which the talents of service providers including conventional medicine vary and can be very problematic if the skill or talent of the healer cannot be quantified in the same way that experience (e.g., number of patients treated) can. The problem is more complicated yet when treatment effectiveness is presumed to depend on a particular relationship, rapport, or bond between the patient and the healer. Unless that relationship or rapport can be defined and assessed at the start of a research trial, there is a risk that a poor outcome will be used as evidence that the necessary relationship did not exist and a good outcome will be used as evidence that it did.

For many CAM therapies, there is a need to pay explicit attention to placebo or expectation effects. In most studies in conventional medicine that include a placebo control arm, the goal of the study is to show that the treatment in question is superior to the placebo. The underlying assumption is that a placebo effect is not real biologically and that the treatment being studied can be deemed to have an effect only if the outcomes that result from the treatment are significantly better than those from the placebo. In many CAM modalities (and in some conventional medicine modalities as well), however, the placebo effect is an inherent part of the mechanism of treatment efficacy. That is, the benefit obtained by the patient is at least partially due to his or her own sense of hope, positive expectation, and activation of self-healing processes. One cannot design a study to eliminate these processes as explanations for outcomes, since they are, by definition within the CAM modality, not a source of noise or confounding but part of the essence of the treatment itself.

In evaluations of CAM therapies, end points may be difficult to measure in a standardized way. The techniques used to measure subjective experiences like pain, fatigue, the ability to perform daily activities, and mood state have experienced significant advances in the past 20 years (IOM, 1999). CAM treatments intended to produce benefits in these areas should be evaluable by using existing, standardized measures with strong scientific foundations.

Other potential outcomes of CAM treatments, however, are not as well defined or measurable. Feelings of general well-being, energy balance, harmony, or centeredness may be harder to measure in a reliable way, and perhaps hard to interpret outside the worldview or belief system of a specific CAM modality. Patients receiving an energy-based CAM therapy, for example, may very well understand questions about energy balance, and reliable and valid measures may be developed in the context of that therapy. The questions may not make as much sense to patients and the measures may not work as well, however, for patients receiving other treatment modalities. It will therefore be difficult to compare scores on such a measure across groups in comparative studies of the energy balance therapy and other CAM or non-CAM therapies. The same problem could hold in reverse, in that quantitative measures of pain intensity, for example, may not make sense and may not have acceptable psychometric properties for patients receiving CAM modalities that do not take a quantitative approach to sensations like pain.

In both CAM and conventional medicine, there are treatments that have some defined boundaries or ranges of acceptable options, as embodied in a training manual, but the healer or provider may have immense room to use variations and his or her own judgment in individual interactions with specific patients. Many psychotherapies, for example, have a general framework and some well-defined features or boundaries, but the specific words used or issues raised at any point in time in a therapy session may differ. These decisions are up to the therapist and are based on a combination of formal training, experience, instinct, and immediate feedback from the patient. It is extremely difficult to study the effectiveness of a specific utterance or even sequence of microlevel interactions between the therapist and the patient, but it may be possible to study the effectiveness of an individual therapist or the approach to therapy taken as a whole. Similarly, in some CAM modalities, it will not be possible to study the effectiveness of a specific maneuver performed in the context of a 30-minute hands-on interaction with a patient (e.g., massage), but it may be possible to evaluate the effectiveness of the approach taken as a whole in comparison with that of some alternative approach to the same problem.

INNOVATIVE STUDY DESIGNS TO ASSESS TREATMENT EFFECTIVENESS OF CAM[1]

Addressing the special challenges mentioned above for research in CAM will require a broadening of thinking about the types of study designs that can produce valid evidence of treatment effectiveness. RCTs and systematic reviews of multiple RCTs will still stand as the "gold standard" of evidence when the key questions have to do with treatment efficacy and when the treatment is amenable to the narrow definition, standardization, and the use of strict controls typical of RCTs. (See Chapter 5 for a discussion of such trials.) When RCTs cannot be done, however, or when the results of RCTs may not be generalizable to the real world of CAM practice, it will be necessary to use other study designs. Some of these options are described in the following sections.

---

[1]This section is largely based on work by Naihua Duan, Joel Braslow, Alison Hamilton Brown, Ted J. Kaptchuk, and Louise E. Tallen in a commissioned paper prepared for the committee's use.

N-of-1 Trials

For some CAM therapies for some patients, it may be possible to organize a series of off-on administrations of a specific therapy. For example, baseline pulmonary function can be tested in patients receiving a homeopathic therapy for hay fever or asthma; and then the therapy can be administered for a period of time, stopped for a period of time and replaced by a placebo, re-administered for a period of time, and so on. Unless the clinician and the patient are both active participants in the essential therapeutic process, both would be blinded as to whether an active treatment or a placebo was given. This may be feasible with many homeopathic or herbal treatments, but it may not be possible with manual manipulation or aromatherapy. The sequence of off and on may also be randomized within and across patients.

Treatments for stable, chronic conditions are best suited to this sort of study, as treatment effectiveness can be determined by the extent to which a defined outcome (seasonal allergies or asthma, in this example) varies with administration of the treatment under study. Inferences are cleanest when a short latency exists between treatment administration and effect and when the treatment has little or no long-lasting effect. When these conditions hold, an N-of-1 trial (a trial with a single subject) can provide strong evidence of the effectiveness of the treatment for that patient. Multiple N-of-1 trials of the same treatment with pooling of the results for adequate numbers of patients can provide the same kind of evidence of effectiveness that would be available through traditional RCTs, assuming that the patients were representative of some larger population to whom the results could be generalized. This approach would be particularly well-suited to CAM therapies that are highly individualized. Each N-of-1 trial, if successful, would provide evidence of the effectiveness of a specific treatment in that one patient; multiple successful trials would provide evidence of the effectiveness of the general concept or manual methods.

Preference RCTs

In most RCTs, patients who agree to participate in the trial also agree to accept randomization to study arms, that is, to active treatment or a placebo treatment. They receive the treatment to which they are randomized, regardless of any preferences that they may have. This kind of study may be difficult to carry out when treatments are already in widespread use, are generally presumed to be effective, or just seem that they should be either more effective or less risky. In these situations a "preference RCT" is appropriate and may also allow the effects of patient preferences on outcomes to be tested empirically.

In a preference RCT (Brewin and Bradley, 1989; McPherson and Britton, 1999; Pocock and Elbourne, 2000), a pool of eligible patients is first asked to indicate whether they have a preference among the treatments being compared. Those who have a preference are given that treatment. Those expressing no preference are randomized to a treatment arm as in a traditional RCT. If the pool of patients is sufficiently large, the design allows three sets of comparisons to be made among the treatments: (1) the effectiveness of different treatments among the randomized patients (which is the same as that in a traditional RCT); (2) the effectiveness of different treatments in those who chose those treatments; and (3) the effectiveness of a specific treatment in those randomized to it compared with the effectiveness in those who chose it. This analysis provides a stronger base from which to make inferences about the effects of treatments in routine daily practice, when patients typically receive a particular treatment on the basis of their preferences.

Wennberg and colleagues (1993) describe a pilot preference RCT in the atricle, Outcomes Research, PORTs, and Health Care Reform. The currently funded NIH Spine Patient Outcomes Research Trial (SPORT), which is in the final stages of recruiting, is another example of this design.

This type of study design may be useful for the study of many CAM modalities for which therapies are widely presumed by practitioners and the lay public to be safe and effective and patients may have existing preferences either for or against a specific therapy.

Observational and Cohort Studies

Observational and cohort studies involve the identification of patients who are eligible for study and who may receive a specified treatment but who may not choose the therapy received as part of the study. Problems with the inferences about effectiveness that can be drawn from observational studies are well known, but in some instances data from these studies may be the only or the best data available. One of the most well-known and recent examples of this comes from the Women's Health Initiative (WHI). In response to observational data that hormone supplements may improve a woman's health peri- and postmenopause, WHI prospectively evaluated the benefits and risks to women of taking hormones during menopause and concluded that the overall health risks exceeded the benefits (Rossouw et al., 2002).

The problems with causal inferences in studies with these designs mainly have to do with the possibility that unmeasured patient characteristics, not balanced by random assignment to treatment, may be the true cause of any effects observed (Little and Rubin, 2000). Methods that can be used to control for measured characteristics (e.g., analysis of covariance, linear regression, and stratification analysis) have been available for many years, but methods that can be used to control for unmeasured characteristics are relatively newer. It is now possible to control for baseline patient characteristics (measured and unmeasured) in better ways by use of analyses like instrumental variable analysis (Hogan and Lancaster, 2004; Newgard et al., 2004; Leigh and Schembri, 2004; Mealli et al., 2004). A detailed discussion of these analytic methods is beyond the charge of this committee, but both methods allow valid causal inferences about treatment effectiveness to be drawn from observational studies.

Case-Control Studies

Other study designs discussed in this chapter are prospective, that is, they identify a pool of eligible patients before treatment is given, and the patients are then monitored through the period of treatment with a series of structured and scheduled measurement instruments. For some questions about CAM treatment effectiveness, however, it may not be possible to mount a reasonable prospective study (for example, if there is no practical way of identifying patients with a defined health problem or identifying and recruiting patients before treatment begins). On the other hand, it may be useful to try to obtain evidence of effectiveness by evaluating data for large numbers of patients who have received the treatment in the past. A case-control study is one example of a study that starts with outcomes and works backwards.

A case-control study involves the identification of people with good or bad health outcomes (e.g., those with a serious illness and those without an illness, those who died of an illness and those who were cured, or those who had relief of chronic pain, and those who did not), and then the assessment of a large number of variables, including the treatments received, to identify the factors correlated with a good or a bad outcome.

The case-control design has a long history in epidemiology and public health; in many instances it is the only effective way of conducting a first inquiry into a presumed cause-effect relationship. The case-control design has important limitations: no matter how detailed and thorough the data collection may be, it is still possible that unknown or unmeasured variables may be the true cause of the differences in outcomes observed and that the relationships observed in the study are not truly causal (Gordis, 1996). Despite its limitations, a case-control study may be an effective way to begin a line of inquiry about treatment effectiveness in CAM, as long as the inquiry continues by use of studies with stronger prospective designs to confirm any presumed causal relationships determined from the findings of the case-control study.

Studies of Bundles or Combinations of Therapies

As mentioned above, it is uncommon for CAM treatments to be given alone, in the sense of either CAM monotherapy or CAM as a strict alternative to traditional medicine. Instead, most patients use a mix of CAM and conventional therapies simultaneously. Studying the effectiveness of one part of a complex mix of treatments is difficult, unless it is possible in the context of a complex study design to vary one part of a package of therapies while the rest of the package is held constant. In most instances, it will be difficult or impossible to isolate the effects of one part of a complex treatment package, but it may be possible to study the effectiveness of the bundle as a whole by using essentially any of the designs described in this section. This will not be fully satisfying to most scientists trained in Western reductionist traditions, but such studies may be adequate to help patients make informed decisions about treatment approaches or for health policymakers or insurance companies to make decisions about coverage and payment.

Some study designs and analytic methods, however, are better suited than others to unraveling the effects of specific parts of a complex treatment package. Observational studies with very large sample sizes can evaluate multiple instances of a large number of specific treatment combinations. They also allow the observation of many complex interactions between patient characteristics and treatment features. The choice of analytic method depends on the presumed underlying mathematics of the combined effects of vectors of patient, provider, treatment, and environmental factors. If these relationships are presumed to be basically linear and additive, then well-known multiple linear regression or logistic regression models can be used to achieve at least a first approximation to the causal relationships in question. A class of methods known as recursive partitioning may be appropriate if the relationships are presumed to be multiplicative or interactive, i.e., the effects of one variable depend on the presence, or value, of one or more other variables, a very likely assumption in many CAM studies in which the interactions among patient characteristics and treatments are presumed to be crucial. Again, a detailed discussion of this is beyond the scope of this report, but well-developed statistical methods, specifically designed to identify the interactive effects of large numbers of causal factors acting simultaneously on a defined outcome variable are available.

Studies of "Manualized" Therapies

Many CAM therapies involve the application of general concepts, theories, or methods but allow for considerable variation in the selection of a specific intervention for a single patient at a single point in time, for example acupuncture and herbal medicine. In most instances this variation is an inherent part of the underlying philosophy of the CAM modality, as it allows the treatment to be tailored to the characteristics of the patient, his or her symptoms, the practitioner, and the time and place of treatment. It is not error or unwanted treatment variability; on the contrary, it may be part of the essence of the CAM approach to be evaluated.

The standardization of treatment characteristic of most clinical research in conventional medicine is therefore inappropriate for studies of these "manualized" therapies that make up part of CAM. By definition and theory, these treatments cannot be standardized in the same way in which drug treatments are standardized by substance, dose, and route and timing of administration. There is precedent for effectiveness research in this domain, however, most notably in psychotherapy (Wampold et al., 1997). In psychotherapy effectiveness research, a model, theory, or general approach is defined and standardized; but the specific utterances by the therapist and the content of interactions between therapist and patient vary.

Effectiveness studies can be conducted on those aspects of the manualized therapies that can be defined and standardized: one general approach versus another approach, one school of thought versus another school of thought, or one intensity or duration of treatment versus another. These studies would be examples of what Tunis et al. (2003) call "practical clinical trials." With some CAM modalities, it may be possible to study the effectiveness of an approach, the school or the intensity of treatment, and the use of a no-treatment or a placebo control as the comparison group. When effectiveness has already been shown relative to the results for the no-treatment controls, studies can be designed to compare more specific features of the general approach or modality.

The designs used for these kinds of studies are not necessarily any different from those used for effectiveness studies in conventional medicine. RCTs, as well as studies with less well-controlled prospective or retrospective designs, may be possible. Statistical methods, outcome measures, sample sizes, and the scope of the conclusions that are drawn may also be essentially the same, because the essence of a typical study would be the comparison of an average outcome and variability in outcomes across two or more groups defined by differences in treatment approaches.

It will not be possible, however, to draw conclusions about any of the specific aspects of treatment that vary without constraint, nor will it be possible to draw conclusions about the effectiveness of an individual provider or therapist unless well-controlled N-of-1 study designs are used in which the individual therapist is the intervention being studied.

Placebo or Expectation Effects

Many CAM modalities include patients' hopes, expectations, emotional states, energies, and other self-healing processes as part of their core "mechanisms of action." Studies of effectiveness of these modalities and therapies cannot consider these factors to be extraneous confounders that are separate from the mechanism(s) of action being tested, as would typically be the case in effectiveness research in conventional medicine.

If the core research question in a CAM effectiveness study involves the identification of a mechanism of action apart from or in addition to nonspecific placebo or expectation effects, then a traditional two-arm study comparing a particular treatment to placebo control would be appropriate. Studies of herbal remedies with inert substances in the control condition or studies of acupuncture with sham-treated controls (Biella et al., 2001) would be examples of this kind of study design. The only CAM therapies or modalities for which this design would not be appropriate would be those that do not claim any mechanism of action other than the patients' own expectations or self-healing processes.

It is also possible to design studies that specifically manipulate the nonspecific placebo or expectation effects to determine whether variation of the "dose" of this variable can influence outcomes. For example, Pollo et al. (2001) conducted a study of how different expectations can produce different analgesic effects. Three groups of patients were treated with buprenorphine, given on request for 3 consecutive days, plus a basal intravenous infusion of saline solution; however each group was given different information about the basal infusions. Group A was told nothing; Group B was told that the infusion was *either* a powerful painkiller or a placebo; and Group C was told that it was a powerful painkiller. The results are shown in Table 4-1.

The investigators concluded that "different verbal instructions about certain and uncertain expectations of analgesia produce different placebo analgesic effects, which in turn, trigger a dramatic change of behavior leading to a significant reduction of opioid intake" (Pollo et al., 2001).

Given that expectation or placebo effects are generally presumed to

TABLE 4-1 Effect of Expectation on Analgesic Effects

Group	Mean Dose (mg) of Buprenorphine Administered
A	1.15 ± 1.14
B	0.91 ± 0.11
C	0.76 ± 0.15

work in a positive direction, it is difficult to imagine an ethically defensible study design in which expectations were specifically manipulated in negative directions (i.e., telling patients that a treatment does not work). Accrual to such a study or the willingness of patients to accept random assignment to a study arm described in that way would presumably be challenging. The ethical and practical limits to manipulation of expectation effects is probably the absence of expectation. Even this limit will be difficult to reach in many studies of CAM effectiveness if the modalities or therapies are widely believed to be effective in the general population.

Even for CAM modalities whose mechanisms of action are largely or exclusively patient expectations or self-healing processes, it may be possible to design studies that compare the relative abilities of two or more modalities to activate those processes and produce measurable health benefits. For example, an ongoing study of patients with irritable bowel syndrome funded by the National Center for Complementary and Alternative Medicine is exploring whether placebo effects (via a sham acupuncture treatment) can be enhanced through variations in patient-provider contexts.

Attribute-Treatment Interaction Analyses

Attribute-treatment interaction analyses is not a study per se but is a way of analyzing data from studies with other designs. A likely result of effectiveness studies in both CAM and conventional medicine, almost regardless of study design, is variability in outcomes among patients within a study and among different studies. This variability leads to questions about reasons for the variability, which can often be expressed by analysis of the subgroups in which the treatments are relatively more or less effective. These analyses are referred to as "attribute-treatment interaction analyses" (Caspi and Bell, 2004a,b).

Because most effectiveness trials are designed with sufficient power to detect differences at the level of the sample as a whole, most subgroup analyses are exploratory in nature, with the conclusions subject to confirmation in more definitive studies conducted later. A variety of statistical methods are available to perform these analyses (for example, see the earlier discussion of recursive partitioning methods); these methods would not be fundamentally different in studies of the effectiveness of CAM than in studies of the effectivenes of conventional medicine. The variables used to classify patients would probably be different, however, since diagnostic and other clinical labels identifying meaningful categories of patients would be different between CAM modalities and conventional medicine and among CAM modalities.

Qualitative Methods

Qualitative methods are not an alternative design to address effectiveness questions but are a way to make better decisions about measurement, sampling, recruitment, and other aspects of a study design. Questions about treatment effectiveness in CAM and in conventional medicine are typically quantitative in nature and involve assessments of more or less of some defined outcome characteristics among patients treated in one way versus another. Evidence for treatment effectiveness in both CAM and conventional medicine therefore typically comes from quantitative studies that use the designs and methods discussed above.

Qualitative research (ethnographic studies, focus groups, and in-depth interviews) cannot generally provide direct evidence of treatment effectiveness because of the relatively small sample sizes, the retrospective versus the prospective nature of participant recruitment and sampling, the absence of random assignment of patients to treatment conditions, and the use of open-ended versus categorical or close-ended data collection formats.

Qualitative research can, however, provide extremely valuable information to help interpret the results of effectiveness studies or to design those studies in the best possible way. Qualitative methods can be used to

- understand the types of patients who use a particular CAM modality, their reasons for using that modality (including perceived effectiveness), and the circumstances or conditions of use;
- understand other treatments that those patients may be using in addition to the specific modality being studied;
- understand patients' and practitioners' definitions of and criteria for treatment effectiveness;
- identify factors that may predict better or worse effectiveness (e.g., different levels of patient expectations and better or worse therapist-patient interactions); and
- understand patients' and providers' models of health and illness and how those models influence CAM use and assessment of treatment effectiveness.

USE OF BOTH TRADITIONAL AND INNOVATIVE STUDY DESIGNS TO CREATE A RICH BODY OF KNOWLEDGE

The committee does not wish to recommend a single study design that is inevitably superior to others or to recommend that studies of treatment effectiveness in CAM always be conducted in a specific way. Alternative study designs have combinations of strengths and weaknesses; the richest information source will be the combined results of studies with several different designs if the strengths of one complement the weaknesses of another. Classic RCTs, for example, will provide strong evidence of cause-and-effect relationships in carefully controlled circumstances, but ideally, the results would be complemented by the results of outcomes or effectiveness studies if the fundamental questions have to do with treatment effectiveness in real-world practice settings (IOM, 1999; Jonas and Linde, 2002).

The use of a variety of study designs to produce a rich, complementary body of evidence for specific treatments or modalities is a desirable approach, but in practice, only limited amounts of money and time are available for effectiveness studies. Study sponsors may have to choose between traditional and innovative study designs, at least at any one point in time, if trials are expensive and budgets are limited.

In those circumstances, trade-offs need to be examined in the context of the question(s) being addressed. If the fundamental question is one of safety, then a surveillance design capable of picking up rare but serious events is indicated. If the therapy is relatively new and unknown and the key questions have to do with efficacy, then a traditional RCT design would fit. If efficacy is accepted but the questions to be addressed have to do with effectiveness across a range of providers and settings, then a large outcomes study aimed at identifying determinants of good and poor outcomes may be indicated. If the key questions have to do with cost-effectiveness, then a more tightly focused outcomes study (i.e., one with fewer patients, providers, or treatment sites) that includes explicit collection of cost data will be required.

RELATIONSHIP BETWEEN BASIC RESEARCH AND CLINICAL RESEARCH

For many treatments, the results of RCTs or other types of clinical studies are the culmination of a much larger sequence of basic research studies that grow out of, contribute to, and increase the understanding of fundamental biological mechanisms of illness. Clinical trials of newer therapies for peptic ulcer, for example, were built on years of basic research on the roles of bacteria and acids in the generation of ulcers. Clinical trials of statins for the treatment of cardiovascular disease were based on years of basic research on the role of cholesterol in cardiovascular disease, and studies of new treatments based on reducing inflammation in coronary arteries will follow basic research on the role of inflammatory processes in the progress from coronary artery disease to acute myocardial infarction.

A crucial synergy exists between basic and clinical research. Basic research seeks to expand knowledge and understanding of the biological mechanisms of illness and treatment. Much of clinical research builds on the results of basic research to determine whether treatments based on new concepts of illness and treatment can produce measurable benefits in defined groups of patients. Findings from clinical research may reinforce the insights gained from basic research or may reveal surprising results that lead to new questions or hypotheses to be tested in laboratory studies. Federal funding agencies (primarily NIH) support a balance of basic and clinical research studies, recognizing that the synergy between the two is crucial to advancing the fundamental science base of medicine. For NIH as a whole, one-third of the funding committed to research is spent on clinical research; for the NIH National Center for Complementary and Alternative Medicine "the ratio of clinical to basic research funding over time was 4:1 in FY 2000, 3:1 in FY 2001, 2.6:1 in FY 2002, 2.5:1 in FY 2003, and will likely fall a little further in 2004" (NCCAM, 2004).

A future strategy for funding CAM research will have to address questions about an appropriate balance between basic and clinical research and related questions about the available infrastructures for both types of studies. For example,

- Should reviewers of proposals for clinical studies in CAM require that there be a foundation of basic research on the underlying mechanisms for the therapy being studied? If so, what must that foundation include? How extensive should it be? Should there be evidence of new insights or breakthroughs, or would it be sufficient for there to be a widely accepted theory (within the relevant provider community) about underlying mechanisms of treatment action?
- Should special requests for proposals be issued for studies of the basic biological mechanisms of specific CAM therapies? If so, for which therapies and which mechanisms should they be issued? Should there be an emphasis on therapies or modalities for which there is significant disagreement about their basic mechanisms in the relevant CAM provider community, or should there be an emphasis on therapies or modalities in which there is general consensus among CAM providers but significant skepticism or lack of understanding of the basic mechanisms among traditional biological scientists?
- If support is given to basic research in CAM, would it be required that the results of the studies have some direct relevance to either current or new CAM treatments, or should support be provided to "knowledge for its own sake"?
- As a condition for funding a body of clinical research on a specific CAM modality, should NIH require some minimum level of ongoing related basic research to expand knowledge of the underlying mechanisms? Or are there CAM modalities for which it would be acknowledged that such basic studies are either unnecessary or impossible to conduct but that clinical studies would be useful nonetheless? In other words, in most clini-

cal studies there is an implicit understanding that a failure of the experimental treatment to produce the expected effect will call into question the assumptions made about the underlying mechanisms and will require the investigators to go back to the drawing board. This may not be the case for some CAM modalities.

• If there is an absence or shortage of existing infrastructure (facilities, trained investigators, or a supportive academic environment) for basic research on an important CAM modality, should the funding strategy emphasize infrastructure development before specific research projects?

CONCEPTUAL MODELS TO GUIDE RESEARCH

Federal agencies supporting research on the effectiveness of CAM therapies may adopt one or more of a variety of conceptual models to guide their decision making about a research agenda and then on the subsequent task of translating research findings into practice guidelines or public policy decisions. The following sections describe several of the possible conceptual models.

Basic Science Excellence

In the basic science excellence model, the highest priority is given to projects that may provide significant breakthroughs in or enhancements of understanding of fundamental biological mechanisms. The concept can be extended to funding decisions about clinical research, in which a conscious choice would be made to fund studies that shed light on underlying mechanisms in preference to those that address only more limited efficacy or effectiveness questions.

Quality of Evidence

In the quality of evidence model, a well-designed study is more important than the ability of a study to shed new light on basic biological processes or mechanisms of treatments. The most important criteria used to make funding decisions are sample size, blinding of study participants, the use of clean methods of data collection and sophisticated methods of data analysis, statistical power, and the clarity of the inferences. An elegant, clean, powerful study addressing a relatively mundane question would be preferred over a less well-designed study addressing a more intriguing question.

Cost-Effectiveness

Cost-effectiveness could actually refer to two different conceptual models. On the one hand, cost-effectiveness could refer to a property of the treatment or CAM modality in question. One could preferentially study CAM modalities with known or expected relatively good cost-effectiveness. Or, one could design studies to assess the cost-effectiveness of a modality or a specific therapy and require that clinical studies include a cost-effectiveness component to be funded. On the other hand, the term could refer to a property of the studies being proposed. A relatively explicit calculation of study cost versus the value of the information to be gained would be done, and only those studies with the best balance would be funded, regardless of other considerations.

Consumer Preference

Consumer preference also has two potential meanings. First, one could design a funding strategy based on the current or potential popularity of CAM modalities or specific treatments. Studies of the most popular or widely used therapies would receive funding preference, under the assumption that it would be more important to gain knowledge of treatment efficacy or effectiveness in those areas than elsewhere. Second, one could preferentially fund studies in which patient preferences would be specifically included. Funding agencies might solicit proposals for preference RCTs so that the results of the studies would perhaps be more generalizable to daily clinical practice, in which patient preferences and expectations are part of the milieu that affects treatment outcomes.

CONCLUSIONS AND RECOMMENDATIONS

This chapter has explored the characteristics of CAM treatments and modalities that make it difficult to apply the traditional RCTs or treatment-effectiveness studies used in conventional medicine. These characteristics include the use of multiple therapies (both CAM and conventional medicine) at the same time, individualization of therapies, the importance of the therapist to the outcome, placebo or expectation effects, the different outcomes valued, and manual treatments. The chapter has also discussed study designs that might be used to address some of these characteristics including N-of-1 trials, preference RCTs, observational and cohort studies, case-control studies, studies of bundles or combinations of therapies, and attribute-treatment interaction analyses. Qualitative research can also help to increase understanding of such things as the types of patients who use particular CAM therapies, their motivations for the use of such therapies, and how they understand health and illness.

The committee believes that it is desirable to use a variety of study designs in the conduct of research of CAM therapies. Given the limited amount of funding available for clinical studies of CAM therapies, decisions about what to evaluate should be made on the basis of one or more of the following criteria. Clearly, no intervention will meet *all* criteria and a therapy should not be excluded from consideration because it does not meet any one particular criterion, for example, biological plausibility. However, the absence of such a mechanism inevitably will raise the level of skepticism about the potential effectiveness of a treatment (whether conventional or CAM) and will increase both the basic research needed to justify funding for clinical studies and the level of evidence from clinical studies needed to consider a treatment as "established."

- A biologically plausible mechanism exists for the intervention but it is recognized that the science base on which plausibility is judged is a work in progress.
- Research could plausibly lead to the discovery of biological mechanisms of disease or treatment effect.
- The condition is highly prevalent (e.g., diabetes mellitus).
- The condition causes a heavy burden of suffering.
- The potential benefit is great.
- Some evidence that the intervention is effective already exists.
- Some evidence that there are safety concerns exists.
- The research design is feasible and research will likely yield an unambiguous result.
- The target condition or the intervention is important enough to have been detected by existing population surveillance mechanisms.

Should CAM be held to the same standards of evidence as conventional medicine? Regardless of the specific choices made about study design, whether it be traditional or innovative, a question that the committee addressed was whether CAM therapies should be held to the same standards of evidence as medications, surgical procedures, or other therapies used in conventional medicine. By the "same standards of evidence," the committee means that an insurance company would require "A-level evidence" (that is, evidence derived from consistent findings from multiple RCTs), for example, to include specific herbal therapies in a pharmacy benefit or formulary if they required A-level evidence for coverage of prescription drugs.

Research on treatment effectiveness is research about cause-effect relationships between the provision of particular treatments and defined pa-

tient outcomes. That is, the hypothesis being tested in effectiveness research is that Treatment *A* produces Health Benefit *Y*. Although CAM and
conventional medicine may differ in terms of the nature of the treatments
provided and the presumed mechanisms by which treatments produce beneficial effects, there is no fundamental diference in the basic nature of either
the cause-effect relationships being tested or the major domains of patient
outcomes being studied. Therefore,

> **The committee recommends that the same principles and standards of
> evidence of treatment effectiveness apply to all treatments, whether
> currently labeled as conventional medicine or CAM. Implementing this
> recommendation requires that investigators use and develop as neces-
> sary common methods, measures, and standards for the generation and
> interpretation of evidence necessary for making decisions about the use
> of CAM and conventional therapies.**

Currently, CAM and conventional medicine are viewed as two separate
sources of ideas to investigate for possible inclusion of therapies in the
evidence-based interventions for comprehensive care. The fact that these
are viewed separately implies that different principles and standards of
evidence are applied. The committee believes that whether the source of an
idea is CAM or whether it is conventional medicine, the same principles
and standards of evidence should apply. There are unproven ideas of all
kinds, both conventional and CAM, which should be studied using a variety of methods. The results of these studies then move the therapies from
unproven ideas to evidence-based practice or comprehensive care.

Chapter 3 of this report discusses three different hierarchies of evidence. Hierarchies of evidence are helpful in making judgments about a
body of evidence and address the public's need for advice about how to
identify better quality studies. Not all CAM modalities are easily amenable
to evaluation, however, and the committee noted, that there are several
considerations involved in applying levels-of-evidence concepts. These
include

• *The importance of carefully defining the treatment or modality being studied.* A given study may be designed to provide evidence on, for
example, the effectiveness of a specific batch of an herbal product, a formu-
lation of that product that is unique to a specific manufacturer but presumably consistent over time, an herb in general (e.g., St. John's wort), or the
whole concept of herbal medicine. In RCTs in conventional medicine, the
treatment or modality being studied is typically very narrowly defined, for
example, a specific dose, timing of administration, and route of administra-

tion of a specific compound. The application of this concept to some CAM modalities in which treatments are tailored may lead to a host of "*N*-of-1" RCTs.

• *The significance of characteristics of the provider as well as the treatment.* Controlled trials of surgical procedures have been done less frequently than studies of medications because it is much more difficult to standardize the process of surgery. Surgery depends to some degree on the skills and training of the surgeon and the specific environment and support team available to the surgeon. A surgical procedure in the hands of a highly skilled, experienced surgeon is different from the same procedure in the hands of an inexperienced and unskilled surgeon (Hu et al., 2003). For many CAM modalities, it is similarly difficult to separate the effectiveness of the treatment from the effectiveness of the person providing the treatment. Indeed, the idea of conceptual separation of treatment and provider would seem foreign for those modalities. The designs of studies of CAM modalities that involve the active participation of a "healer" must incorporate the characteristics of that person as well as the characteristics of the treatment being applied by that person.

• *Different underlying theoretical and diagnostic systems.* Concepts of levels of evidence and evidence-based medicine in conventional medicine rely on a generally accepted diagnostic classification system that is embodied in formal diagnostic systems like the International Classification of Diseases-Version 10 (ICD-10) and the Diagnostic and Statistical Manual-Version IV (DSM-IV). It will be somewhat challenging to apply similar study designs, measures of clinical endpoints, and standards of evidence to therapies that use different diagnostic systems and therefore to identify different sets of patients as the group to whom the study results apply. It will be even more challenging to apply these concepts to any CAM modalities that emphasize the uniqueness of each individual patient and that patient's complex of symptoms and to avoid diagnostic classifications entirely.

• *Endpoints like feelings of emotional or spiritual well-being that are difficult to measure.* The most important dependent variables in many CAM modalities will be hard to define in objective terms and may vary from patient to patient (Jonas and Linde, 2002). A study of whether acupuncture is effective for patients with cancer may not be able to focus on mortality or shrinkage of tumors but, instead may have to focus on questions of whether the patients feel relief of pain and other symptoms and whether they feel more in control of their illness and are better able to manage the cancer along with their other daily tasks.

• *Difficult or impossible to conduct double-blind trials with some modalities.* The concept of blinding in which the patients and the treating clinicians participating in clinical trials do not know what treatment the patient is receiving is an important way to minimize expectation effects and biases on the part of both the patient and the clinician. For most CAM modalities, however, blinding is very difficult or impossible.

A CAM research portfolio with a variety of types of studies will provide a great deal of knowledge about the use of CAM therapies by the American public. The next chapter discusses what is known about efficacies of some CAM therapies, identifies existing gaps, and proposes a framework that can be used to conduct research on CAM.

REFERENCES

Biella G, Sotgiu ML, Pellegata G, Paulesu E, Castiglioni I, Fazio F. 2001. Acupuncture produces central activations in pain regions. *Neuroimage* 14(1 Pt 1):60–66.

Brewin CR, Bradley C. 1989. Patient preferences and randomised clinical trials. *BMJ* 299(6694):313–315.

Caspi O, Bell IR. 2004a. One size does not fit all: Aptitude-Treatment Interaction (ATI) as a conceptual framework for CAM outcome research. Part I. What is ATI research? *J Altern Complement Med* 10(3).

Caspi O, Bell IR. 2004b. One size does not fit all: Aptitude-Treatment Interaction (ATI) as a conceptual framework for CAM outcome research. Part II. Research designs and their applications. *J Altern Complement Med* 10(4).

Eisenberg DM, Kessler RC, Foster C, Norlock FE, Calkins DR, Delbanco TL. 1993. Unconventional medicine in the United States: Prevalance, costs, and patterns of use. *N Engl J Med* 328(4):246–252.

Eisenberg DM, Davis RB, Ettner SL, Appel S, Wilkey S, Van Rompay M, Kessler RC. 1998. Trends in alternative medicine use in the United States, 1990-1997: Results of a follow-up national survey. *JAMA* 280(18):1569–1575.

Gordis L. 1996. *Epidemiology*. Philadelphia, PA: W.B. Saunders Company.

Hogan JW, Lancaster T. 2004. Instrumental variables and inverse probability weighting for causal inference from longitudinal observational studies. *Stat Methods Med Res* 13(1): 17–48.

Hu JC, Gold KF, Pashos CL, Mehta SS, Litwin MS. 2003. Role of surgeon volume in radical prostatectomy outcomes. *J Clin Oncol* 21(3):401–405.

IOM (Institute of Medicine). 1999. *Gulf War Veterans: Measuring Health*. Washington, DC: National Academy Press.

Jonas WB, Linde K. 2002. Conducting and Evaluating Clinical Research on Complementary and Alternative Medicine. In: Gallin JI, ed. *Principles and Practice of Clinical Research*. San Diego, CA: Academic Press. Pp. 401–426.

Krieger D. 1998. Dolores Krieger, RN, PhD healing with therapeutic touch. Interview by Bonnie Horrigan. *Altern Ther Health Med* 4(1):86–92.

Leigh JP, Schembri M. 2004. Instrumental variables technique: Cigarette price provided better estimate of effects of smoking on SF-12. *J Clin Epidemiol* 57(3):284–293.

Little RJ, Rubin DB. 2000. Causal effects in clinical and epidemiological studies via potential outcomes: Concepts and analytical approaches. *Annu Rev Public Health* 21:121–145.

McPherson K, Britton A. 1999. The impact of patient treatment preferences on the interpretation of randomised controlled trials. *Eur J Cancer* 35(11):1598–1602.

Mealli F, Imbens GW, Ferro S, Biggeri A. 2004. Analyzing a randomized trial on breast self-examination with noncompliance and missing outcomes. *Biostatistics* 5(2):207–222.

NCCAM (National Center for Complementary and Alternative Medicine). 2004. *National Center for Complementary and Alternative Medicine: The First Five Years*. Bethesda, MD: National Institutes of Health.

Newgard CD, Hedges JR, Arthur M, Mullins RJ. 2004. Advanced statistics: The propensity score—a method for estimating treatment effect in observational research. *Acad Emerg Med* 11(9):953–961.

Park CM. 2002. Diversity, the individual, and proof of efficacy: Complementary and alternative medicine in medical education. *Am J Public Health* 92(10):1568–1572.

Pocock SJ, Elbourne DR. 2000. Randomized trials or observational tribulations? *N Engl J Med* 342(25):1907–1909.

Pollo A, Amanzio M, Arslanian A, Casadio C, Maggi G, Benedetti F. 2001. Response expectancies in placebo analgesia and their clinical relevance. *Pain* 93(1):77–84.

Rossouw JE, Anderson GL, Prentice RL, LaCroix AZ, Kooperberg C, Stefanick ML, Jackson RD, Beresford SA, Howard BV, Johnson KC, Kotchen JM, Ockene J. 2002. Risks and benefits of estrogen plus progestin in healthy postmenopausal women: Principal results from the Women's Health Initiative randomized controlled trial. *JAMA* 288(3):321–333.

Tunis SR, Stryer DB, Clancy CM. 2003. Practical clinical trials: Increasing the value of clinical research for decision making in clinical and health policy. *JAMA* 290(12):1624–1632.

Wampold BE, Mondin GW, Moody M, Stich F, Benson K, Ahn H. 1997. A meta-analysis of outcome studies comparing bona fide psychotherapies: Empiricially, "all must have prizes." *Psychol Bull* 122(3):203–215.

Wennberg JE, Barry MJ, Fowler FJ, Mulley A. 1993. Outcomes research, PORTs, and health care reform. *Ann NY Acad Sci* 703:52–62.

Wolsko PM, Eisenberg DM, Davis RB, Ettner SL, Phillips RS. 2002. Insurance coverage, medical conditions, and visits to alternative medicine providers: Results of a national survey. *Arch Intern Med* 162(3):281–287.

5

State of Emerging Evidence on CAM

For policy makers, practitioners, patients, and health care system managers to make informed decisions about the use of complementary and alternative (CAM) therapies, they must have both access to and a means of evaluating the results of research on the topic. This chapter discusses the evidence that forms the basis for such decision making and the methods of evaluation, as well as the available resources providing access to the results of existing research on CAM interventions.

In CAM as well as in conventional medicine, randomized controlled trials (RCTs), when possible, are the preferable study design for assessing efficacy. RCTs use random allocation to create comparable groups, after which an intervention is introduced. This intervention consists of treatment for the test group and a placebo, no treatment, or another active treatment for the control group. Once the outcome is recorded, any observable differences between the treatment and control group should be attributable to the intervention because the groups were initially comparable before the intervention was introduced.

A systematic review uses explicit, systematic methods to review existing research, particularly the effectiveness of health care interventions, as evaluated by RCTs. Some systematic reviews may include meta-analyses, which provide an overview of the results of similar studies by the use of statistical methods to evaluate the data from many studies. Systematic reviews are widely considered the best method for gathering and synthesizing evidence as well as for determining gaps that exist in current research. Although basic science research and evaluation of cost-effectiveness are also important aspects of research on CAM therapies and modalities, the focus of the following sections is the evaluation of the clinical efficacies of therapies by RCTs and systematic reviews.

SOURCES OF INFORMATION ON HIGH-QUALITY EVIDENCE

Two main sources of information about published RCTs and systematic reviews are *The Cochrane Library* and MEDLINE. Critical reviews of reviews and Agency for Healthcare Research and Quality (AHRQ) Evidence Reports summarize the information by using rigorous and objective methods. National Institutes of Health (NIH) Consensus Statements incorporate evidence from RCTs and systematic reviews together with the judgments of a panel of nonadvocate, nongovernmental experts, to reach a decision about the efficacy and safety of a particular treatment.

MEDLINE

MEDLINE, a product of the National Library of Medicine, is an extensive bibliographic database covering all areas of clinical medicine and biomedical research. The bibliographic citations and abstracts indexed in MEDLINE are from more than 4,600 biomedical journals published worldwide, and the database includes information on all randomized trials in MEDLINE-indexed journals, regardless of the methodological quality or clinical relevance. MEDLINE is accessible online and is free of charge to the public, and most of its 12 million citations are available in English, at least as abstracts. The database includes studies published since 1966, the year that MEDLINE began, and is updated on a regular basis (National Library of Medicine, 2002).

In recent years, relevant indexing terms have been introduced on MEDLINE to facilitate queries on trials and systematic reviews related to CAM. MEDLINE introduced the publication type "randomized controlled trial" for specific RCTs in 1991 and the subject subset "systematic review" in 2001. The subject subset "CAM" was introduced in 2001 and includes all records identified through the execution of a complex, highly sensitive search strategy designed to identify all records in the MEDLINE database related to CAM. The introduction of these terms allows interested individuals to make simple queries of MEDLINE to estimate changes in the evidence base for CAM from the results of RCTs and systematic reviews over time. Figure 5-1 charts the tremendous growth in the number of RCTs over the past 20 years, and Figure 5-2 shows that the rate of increase of reviews and meta-analyses is even greater. These increases parallel general trends of growth in trials and meta-analyses over the past twenty years (Lee et al., 2001). Despite these developments, however, limitations of MEDLINE persist: not all studies in MEDLINE are indexed with the appropriate terms

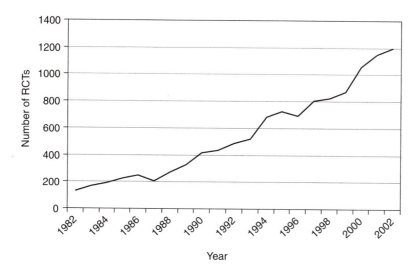

FIGURE 5-1 Number of CAM RCTs indexed on MEDLINE, 1982 to 2002. This search was performed on December 11, 2003, by using a search strategy with the following terms to obtain counts for each year: randomized controlled trial (publication type) AND year (publication date).

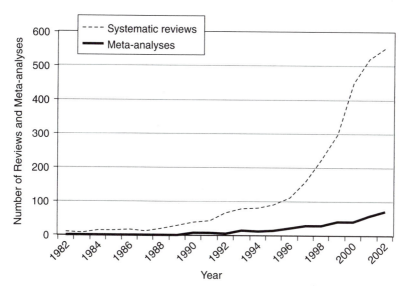

FIGURE 5-2 Number of reviews and meta-analyses related to CAM indexed on MEDLINE, 1982 to 2002. This search was performed on December 11, 2003, by using a search strategy with the following two sets of terms to obtain counts for each year: systematic (subset type) AND year (publication date) and meta-analysis (publication type) AND year (publication date).

(Dickersin et al., 1994), and many reports, especially in the field of CAM, are not included on MEDLINE (Egger et al., 2003).

The Cochrane Library

The Cochrane Library, unique both for its scope and for its methodological standards, is supported through the work of the Cochrane Collaboration (Dickersin and Manheimer, 1998), an international organization of more than 9,000 contributors (mostly volunteers) from more than 80 countries (Allen and Clarke, 2003). The Cochrane Complementary Medicine Field, based at the University of Maryland Center for Integrative Medicine, coordinates all of the CAM-related activities of the Cochrane Collaboration, including the development of a database with information on more than 7,000 controlled trials of CAM therapies and modalities, and facilitates the preparation of CAM reviews and the promotion of these reviews, especially among the members of the CAM community.

Members of the Cochrane Collaboration prepare up-to-date, reliable summaries or systematic reviews of every kind of health care therapy. Cochrane reviews, which are intended to answer questions about health care and to guide providers in practical decision making about treatment, are published quarterly in *The Cochrane Library*. Although reviews of journal articles are current only as of their date of publication, the electronic format of *The Cochrane Library* allows the reviews to be updated easily and periodically to account for new evidence. In addition, Cochrane reviews have shown greater methodological rigor than systematic reviews and meta-analyses published in paper-based journals (Jadad et al., 1998, 2000). The use of rigorous methods is also ensured by the requirement that the protocols used for a review be prepared before a review is conducted and by an extensive system of peer review.

Because the information in *The Cochrane Library* is prescreened to a certain extent and includes only studies evaluating health care therapies, it is of generally higher quality and greater relevance to patient care than the information available on MEDLINE. The Cochrane Database of Systematic Reviews and the Cochrane Central Register of Controlled Trials comprise the major databases of the Cochrane Collaboration. If no review is available on the Cochrane Database of Systematic Reviews, one can check *The Cochrane Library's* Database of Abstracts of Reviews of Effectiveness (a database of reviews collected by the Cochrane Collaboration but not prepared according to the strict standards of Cochrane reviews) or the applicable trials registered with the Cochrane Central Register of Controlled Trials.

The Cochrane database of CAM-related clinical trials is an immensely valuable resource because it covers many of the controlled trials that would not be included on MEDLINE. Vickers (1998) analyzed the Cochrane register for studies related to CAM and found that 19 percent of the citations were not indexed on MEDLINE. The trials included in the register were derived from 965 different journals; 84 percent of the trials were published in conventional medical journals. The numbers of trials per therapy varied a great deal: although Vickers found 554 trials of acupuncture and 804 of herbal medicine, he retrieved only 47 trials of aromatherapy. The number of trials per condition also varied, with 501 trials of cardiovascular disease, 386 trials of musculoskeletal disorders, and 293 trials of surgery-related symptoms, but only 11 trials of fatigue disorders. The objective of the register is to include all large multicenter trials, such as those recently published showing that St. John's wort and echinacea are ineffective for the treatment of major depression and the common cold, respectively (Hypericum Depression Trial Study Group, 2002; Taylor et al., 2003). Also included are smaller RCTs, such as pilot studies of acupuncture conducted in China. The ultimate aim of developing the Cochrane CAM register is to provide a comprehensive source of trials of CAM therapies and modalities, thus reducing the need for systematic reviewers and others to search multiple sources.

At present *The Cochrane Library* contains 145 CAM-related systematic and an additional 340 non-Cochrane CAM-related systematic reviews (see Table 5-1 for a sampling of therapies covered by Cochrane and non-Cochrane reviews). These reviews cover many areas of CAM, with particular strength in the fields of acupuncture and herbal medicine, reflecting not only the large number of trials in these fields, but also the great interest of clinicians, policy makers, and consumers in these areas.

There are some disparities between evidence from Cochrane reviews and evidence from clinical practice. For example, although relaxation techniques (e.g., meditation) are the most commonly used CAM therapy among the U.S. general population (Eisenberg et al., 1998) and the fourth most commonly used therapy in hospital-based CAM or wellness centers (Health Forum, 2003), few Cochrane reviews have evaluated such therapies. On the other hand, although herbal therapy and treatment with other dietary supplements are not widely offered in U.S. hospitals, they are the most reviewed and are among the therapies that are the most commonly used by the U.S. public (Eisenberg et al., 1998).

The international structure of the Cochrane Collaboration plays a critical role in the identification of CAM trials and the preparation of reviews of CAM treatments and modalities because the therapies considered CAM in the United States are often the traditional medicines used by the populations of other countries. Through the work of the 14 Cochrane Centers worldwide, journals published around the world are hand searched to identify RCTs on conventional medicine therapies and CAM therapies and

TABLE 5-1 Number of Cochrane and Non-Cochrane Reviews, by Therapy, March 2004

Therapy	Cochrane Reviews	Non-Cochrane Reviews
Acupuncture	10	69
Alexander technique	1	0
Art therapy	1	1
Biofeedback	2	26
Chiropractic	2	33
Dietary supplements (nonherbal)	71	46
Electromagnetic therapy	3	11
Herbal therapy	23	79
Homeopathy	4	34
Laser therapy	4	4
Massage therapy	4	18
Prayer	1	2
Transcutaneous electrical nerve stimulation	7	11
Therapeutic touch	1	3
Yoga	2	4
Other	27	91

NOTE: Some reviews cover multiple therapies and are therefore counted multiple times. The total number of Cochrane and Non-Cochrane reviews represented in this table are 156 and 340, respectively.

modalities that may be relevant and eligible for a systematic review. The Chinese Cochrane Centre, for example, has identified an estimated 10,000 trials of traditional Chinese medicine through their hand searches (Tang and Wong, 1998); moreover, dozens of reviews of traditional Chinese medicine are under way.

Cochrane Review Evidence for CAM[1]

All Cochrane reviews, be they of CAM or conventional medicine therapies, apply the same standards, that is, therapies within both categories are

---

[1]The committee did not include information about the general direction of effect for the AHRQ reports because the individual reports covered too wide a range of conditions (e.g., S-Adenosyl-L-Methionine (SAMe) for Depression, Osteoarthritis, and Liver Disease) and therapies (e.g., Mind-Body Interventions for Gastrointestinal Conditions). Cochrane reviews, in contrast, typically evaluate a specific therapy for a specific condition. Concise summaries of the findings of each of the AHRQ Technology Reports are presented on the AHRQ website or http://www.ahrq.gov/clinic/epcindex.htm#complementary.

evaluated according to the strength of evidence from RCTs. To evaluate the evidence for CAM from Cochrane reviews, all reviews of CAM-related therapies were selected from *The Cochrane Library* and assigned categories, as described below. As a means of applying an objective, reproducible, and operational eligibility criterion, the committee considered Cochrane reviews to be related to CAM only if the therapies reviewed were listed as therapies in the National Center for Complementary and Alternative Medicine (NCCAM)-National Library of Medicine CAM on PubMed, a database of abstracts and articles on CAM-related therapies. The database can be accessed by use of a multipage search strategy designed to identify all studies listed on PubMed that should be indexed in the PubMed CAM subset. The results from all eligible Cochrane reviews of CAM therapies were assigned to one of the following six categories by two trained methodologists: positive effect, possibly positive effect, two active treatments are equal, insufficient or inconclusive evidence of an effect, no effect, or harmful effect. When the two raters differed on their classification of the treatment described in a review, a third rater trained in RCT and systematic review methodologies assigned the final classification. This rating system was used in a previous study to assess the evidence base for conventional medicine according to the information found in Cochrane reviews (Ezzo et al., 2001).

The agreement of the classification assignment between the initial two raters was 83 percent. For the 17 percent of reviews for which the initial raters assigned different classification codes, the third rater agreed with one of the initial two raters' codes in all cases. The largest number of treatments described in the reviews were classified as insufficient evidence of an effect (n = 82; 56.6 percent), followed by positive effect (n = 36; 24.8 percent) and possibly positive effect (n = 18; 12.4 percent). Only one review described a treatment that was classified as harmful (Caraballoso et al., 2003) (see Table 5-2). The reviews describing treatments classified as having positive effects are listed in Table 5-3. Although this exercise suggests that there is strong evidence for the effectiveness of some CAM therapies, much more research is required, as demonstrated by the large proportion of reviews of treatments classified as insufficient evidence of an effect. The fact that only one of the treatments in the Cochrane reviews fell into the harmful effect category suggests that clinical trials of CAM therapies have posed little risk to the participants.

Some interesting findings emerge when the results of the evaluation of Cochrane reviews of CAM therapies are compared with the results of the earlier study (Ezzo et al., 2001) evaluating Cochrane reviews of conventional therapies: insufficient evidence of an effect was determined for a larger proportion of CAM therapies (56.6 percent for CAM versus 21.3

TABLE 5-2 Conclusion Categories, Definitions, and Proportions Classified by Readers for Cochrane CAM Reviews

Conclusion Category	Definition	Readers' Consensual Rating for Included Reviews ($n = 145$) (%)
Positive effect	Treatment is more beneficial/effective than control for the primary outcome.	36 (24.8)
Possibly positive effect	Treatment may have a positive effect, but a major unresolved methodological issue, such as all studies being very low quality, or findings based on only one study, precludes making a definitive statement.	18 (12.4)
Two active treatments are equal	Two biologically active treatments, such as two antibiotics, are equally as effective for the condition being treated. This category to be used only when comparing two active treatments, not placebo or no treatment.	1 (.6)
Insufficient/ inconclusive evidence	There is not sufficient evidence to determine effectiveness.	82 (56.6)
No effect	There is sufficient evidence, and there is no effect.	7 (4.8)
Harmful effect	Treatment does more harm than good.	1 (.6)

percent for conventional medicine), CAM therapies were less likely to be classified as harmful (8.1 percent for conventional medicine versus 0.69 percent for CAM) or as having no effect (20.0 percent for conventional medicine versus 4.8 percent for CAM), and classification of the therapies as having positive or a possibly positive effect was approximately equal for CAM and conventional medicine therapies (41.3 percent for conventional medicine versus 38.4 percent for CAM). In making comparisons between the two studies, however, it is important to keep in mind that the studies were conducted at different times and thus included different sets of Cochrane reviews. The study of Ezzo et al. (2001) included only those reviews published in *The Cochrane Library* at the time of its first issue in 1998, whereas the analysis of CAM described above included reviews published in the 2004 issue of the database, which is now much more comprehensive and better developed.

TABLE 5-3 Cochrane CAM Reviews[a] with Positive Effects

Study	Therapy	Indication[b]	Limitation/ Comment[c]
Atallah AN et al., 2004	Calcium	Preventing hypertensive disorders and related problems in pregnancy	1, 4
Beckles WN et al., 2004	Omega-3 fatty acids (from fish oil)	Cystic fibrosis	1, 2
Brosseau L et al., 2004	Transcutaneous electrical nerve stimulation (TENS)	Rheumatoid arthritis in the hand	1
D'Souza RM and D'Souza R, 2004	Vitamin A	Measles	4
Darlow B and Austin N, 2004	Selenium	Short-term morbidity in preterm neonates	4
Darlow BA and Graham PJ, 2004	Vitamin A	Preventing morbidity and mortality in very low-birthweight infants	1, 4
Douglas RM et al., 2004	Vitamin C	Preventing and treating the common cold	1 (does not prevent colds; only reduces duration of symptoms)
Evans JR, 2004	Antioxidant vitamin and mineral supplements	Age-related macular degeneration	4, 5
Farmer A et al., 2004	Fish oil	Type 2 diabetes mellitus	3, 5
Furlan AD et al., 2004	Massage	Low back pain	2, 6
Herxheimer A and Petrie KJ, 2004	Melatonin	Preventing and treating jet lag	5

continued

TABLE 5-3 Continued

Study	Therapy	Indication[b]	Limitation/ Comment[c]
Homik J et al., 2004	Calcium and vitamin D	Corticosteroid-induced osteoporosis	—
Howlett A and Ohlsson A, 2004	Inositol	Respiratory distress syndrome in preterm infants	—
Hulme J et al., 2004	Electromagnetic fields	Osteoarthritis	—
Jepson RG et al., 2004	Cranberries	Preventing urinary tract infections	1
Linde K and Mulrow CD, 2004	St. John's wort	Depression	2
Little CV and Parsons T, 2004	Herbal therapy	Osteoarthritis	—(only one herb found effective)
Lumley J et al., 2004	Periconceptual supplementation with folate and/or multivitamins	Preventing neural tube defects	4
Mahomed K, 2004	Folate supplementation in pregnancy	Biochemical parameters and pregnancy outcome	3, 4
Mahomed K, 2004	Iron and folate supplementation in pregnancy	Biochemical parameters and pregnancy outcome	3, 4
Mahomed K, 2004	Iron supplementation in pregnancy	Biochemical parameters and pregnancy outcome	3, 4
Melchart D et al., 2004	Acupuncture	Headache	—
Melchart D et al., 2004	Echinacea	Preventing and treating the common cold	1
Ortiz Z et al., 2004	Folic acid and folinic acid	Reducing side effects in patients receiving methotrexate	1

TABLE 5-3 Continued

Study	Therapy	Indication[b]	Limitation/ Comment[c]
Osiri M et al., 2004	TENS	Knee osteoarthritis	1
Pittler MH and Ernst E, 2004	Horse chestnut	Chronic venous insufficiency	—
Pittler MH and Ernst E, 2004	Kava	Anxiety	5
Proctor ML et al., 2004	TENS and acupuncture	Primary dysmenorrhoea	1
Shea B et al., 2004	Calcium	Bone loss	—
Taylor MJ et al., 2004	Folate	Depression	4
Towheed TE et al., 2004	Glucosamine	Osteoarthritis	1, 2
Wilson ML and Murphy PA, 2004	Herbal and dietary therapies	Primary and secondary dysmenorrhoea	—
Wilt T et al., 2004	African prune	Benign prostatic hyperplasia	1, 2
Wilt T et al., 2004	Beta-sitosterols	Benign prostatic hyperplasia	2
Wilt T et al., 2004	Saw palmetto	Benign prostatic hyperplasia	2
Wilt T et al., 2004	Cernilton	Benign prostatic hyperplasia	1, 2, 6

[a]Our application of the list of terms used in the CAM on PubMed search strategy in defining our eligibility criteria for *CAM-related* resulted in the inclusion in our sample of some Cochrane reviews that many would not consider to be CAM-related. It is notoriously difficult to make the determination of whether or not a therapy should be considered CAM-related, and this decision must often be made in the context of the therapy's application (e.g., for nutrients, whether it is used as a supplement or to address a deficiency); the setting in which the therapy is used (e.g., hospital, self-care); the current state of the evidence for the therapy (e.g., a therapy such as folic acid for neural tube defects has strong supportive evidence which has resulted in its integrated into the health care system); and the point of historical time at which the evaluation of the therapy as CAM or not CAM is made. Our CAM eligibility criteria, while initially deemed the most objective and reproducible approach

continued

TABLE 5-3 Continued

Study	Therapy	Indication[b]	Limitation/ Comment[c]

for selecting CAM reviews, does not take into account the indication for which the therapy is used and has resulted in our including multiple reviews that are not CAM (e.g., vitamin A for measles) and excluding other reviews that are CAM (e.g., speleotherapy for the treatment of asthma), but the therapy reviewed is not a term in the CAM on PubMed search strategy. Because indexing reports always involves some degree of subjectivity (especially when indexing on a difficult-to-pin-down term such as CAM) and because the CAM on PubMed search strategy still requires improvements in the recall and precision of its terms, a second review, by an authority in the field, of reviews that were possibly inappropriately included or excluded based on the strict application of the CAM on PubMed search strategy terms, may be necessary.

[b]Indication is for the treatment of the condition unless specifically listed as prevention

[c]1= Optimal dosage, preparation, or method of administration needs further investigation

2= Long-term effectiveness data lacking

3= Effects only demonstrated on blood marker surrogate outcome measures

4= Results may only apply to populations with low intake of nutrient

5= May be possible adverse effects in some people, according to either the review data or other research

6= These reviews found positive effects in comparison to both active and inactive controls; for all others, positive effects were in comparison with inactive controls

Sufficiently powered, well-designed RCTs of adequate duration may be necessary to confirm the positive conclusions of these Cochrane reviews.

Ongoing Trials

An often cited limitation of the systematic review is that it is generally restricted to published RCTs; if the published RCTs are not representative of all RCTs undertaken (i.e., both published and unpublished RCTs), the review may be unreliable (Manheimer and Anderson, 2002). Although various groups have tried to identify, organize, and disseminate information on unpublished and ongoing RCTs, much work remains to be done. One attempt to bridge the information gap is the website Current Controlled Trials (http://www. controlled-trials.com), an international resource providing metadata about registers of controlled trials in a searchable database. Government agencies also compile registers: the NCCAM website contains a list of NCCAM-funded clinical trials, whereas ClinicalTrials. gov provides access to a database of thousands of clinical studies being sponsored by NIH, other federal agencies, and the pharmaceutical industry. However, none of these resources is comprehensive at this time; only a comprehensive register of all ongoing CAM trials would allow researchers to know which CAM-related RCTs have been conducted, regardless of whether results are available.

Summarizing the Reviews

In recent years, many systematic reviews of CAM therapies have been conducted and efforts are under way to synthesize and summarize as comprehensively as possible the evidence available from these reviews.

Systematic Reviews of Reviews

One way in which data are synthesized is through systematic reviews of reviews, which provide an overview of a therapy's effectiveness across all conditions. It is important to note that those preparing the summary must be aware of and acknowledge or adjust for the fact that some studies may appear in more than one review of a given topic.

Reviews of reviews use comprehensive searches, strict inclusion criteria, and data extraction with pretested forms. These reviews of reviews summarize the basic information from individual reviews, including conditions, interventions, methodological features, and results, as well as present the number of studies reviewed and the reviewers' own conclusions (Linde et al., 2001a,c,d).

AHRQ Evidence Reports

AHRQ, the leading federal agency concerned with research on health care quality, efficiency, effectiveness, and safety, prepares evidence reports and technology assessments that provide information on the clinical efficacies of medical interventions on the basis of systematic reviews and, when appropriate, meta-analyses. Many AHRQ evidence reports relate to CAM interventions (Table 5-4).

NIH Consensus Statement

An NIH consensus statement is prepared by a panel of experts who review key questions and data about various therapies before an audience that comprises other experts in various medical fields. The panel, working with this audience of experts, addresses a predefined question and reaches conclusions on the basis of both the scientific data presented to the panel and data from the relevant literature gathered from MEDLINE. In 1997, NIH produced a consensus statement on acupuncture and concluded that, despite equivocal results in many studies, acupuncture is clearly effective for postoperative dental care and the prevention of nausea and vomiting in adults after surgery and chemotherapy and is possibly effective for many other conditions (National Institutes of Health, 1998). Nevertheless, poor study designs, inadequate sample sizes, and other problems invalidated the

TABLE 5-4 CAM Evidence Reports and Technology Assessments[a] of the U.S. Agency for Health Care Research and Quality[b] (as of January 2004)

Title	Year of Publication
Acupuncture for fibromyalgia	2003
Acupuncture for osteoarthritis	2003
Antioxidant supplements, prevention and treatment of cancer	2003
Antioxidant supplements, prevention and treatment of cardiovascular disease	2003
Ayurvedic interventions for diabetes mellitus: A systematic review	2001
Ephedra and ephedrine for weight loss and athletic performance enhancement: Clinical efficacy of and side effects	2003
Garlic: Effects on cardiovascular risks and disease, protective effects against cancer, and clinical adverse effects	2000
Milk thistle: Effects on liver disease and cirrhosis and clinical adverse effects	2000
Mind-body interventions for gastrointestinal conditions	2001
S-Adenosyl-L-Methionine (SAMe) for depression, osteoarthritis, and liver disease	2002

[a]Evidence Reports and Technology Assessments are based on a comprehensive review of the literature, together with rigorous qualitative, and as appropriate, quantitative methods of synthesizing data from multiple studies.

[b]Full versions of these reports, as well as brief summaries, are available through the AHRQ website (www.ahrq.gov).

results of many studies, as did problems with the inclusion of appropriate controls. The NIH consensus statement recommended further research, as future studies will probably discover additional therapeutic uses for acupuncture.

Although systematic reviews are not themselves meant to function as recommendations or guidelines, they should ideally form the basis for guideline creation. Governments and medical institutions may adopt various methods of summarizing reviews and translating the findings from those reviews into recommendations for use by clinicians (Grol and Grimshaw, 2003; Shekelle et al., 2001; Shiffman et al., 2003; Silagy et al., 2001). Such organizations must also evaluate the economic costs of CAM therapies, as well as their efficacies, when deciding whether or not to offer them to patients (Friedman et al., 1995; Lorig et al., 1999). A recent systematic review of economic analyses of CAM therapies showed that, for the most part, "there is a paucity of rigorous studies that could provide conclusive evidence of differences in costs and outcomes between CAM therapies and orthodox medicine" (White and Ernst, 2000).

Evaluating Study Quality

Importance of Quality

As the discussion above makes clear, a substantial base of information comprising the results of RCTs and systematic reviews evaluating the effectiveness of CAM therapies now exists. The quality of these studies varies however, and the lower-quality RCTs have exaggerated CAM treatment effects (Juni et al., 2001; Schulz et al., 1995). Thus, the evaluation of study quality is of utmost importance to determine the validity of study results. Quality evaluations, already well under way in conventional medicine, are important to ensure the validity and quality of the research and should therefore become standard practice in CAM as well. To address this important issue, researchers have begun devising methods for the optimal conduct of RCTs of CAM therapies, as well as for evaluation of the quality of the research already conducted.

Important Components of Quality

Because quality varies across studies and it was found in RCTs of conventional medicine therapies that lower-quality RCTs have exaggerated treatment effects (Juni et al., 2001; Schulz et al., 1995), it is important to establish standards for evaluation. Study quality can be evaluated by various strategies, but any instrument used to evaluate quality must take into account randomization, blinding, dropouts, and allocation concealment. For example, the Jadad Scale (Jadad et al., 1996) evaluates the quality of reporting by asking a variety of questions: Was the study described as randomized? Was the study described as double-blind? Was there a description of the study participants who withdrew and dropped out? These questions help to ascertain whether the conduct and reporting of the trial are adequate. It is also important that RCTs have a sample size large enough to determine the effectiveness of the intervention. Systematic reviews are evaluated on the basis of whether they undertake a comprehensive literature search with unambiguous inclusion and exclusion criteria for studies, as well as on the basis of whether they use explicit and transparent methods to evaluate and summarize study data.

Methodological Quality of CAM-Related RCTs

The research conducted thus far tends to show not only that RCTs of CAM have significant shortcomings and omissions both in the methodology and in the reporting but also that the quality of CAM-related RCTs is inconsistent (Linde et al., 2001b). For example, larger trials included on MEDLINE and published in English are, in general, of higher quality than those harder-to-find trials not published in English (Egger et al., 2003; Linde et al., 2001a,c,d). Most trials of homeopathy, herbal medicine, and acupuncture had major problems with their reporting and the study methodology, such as the documentation of allocation concealment, dropouts, and withdrawals. These shortcomings also varied by intervention (Linde et al., 2001b).

Efforts to Improve Quality

Many efforts are under way to improve the quality of trials and systematic reviews, including the establishment of CONSORT, QUOROM, and STRICTA (Standards for Reporting Interventions in Controlled Trials of Acupuncture) guidelines. The CONSORT statement helps to improve the quality of RCTs by providing a checklist and flow diagram against which the trial procedures can be measured, as well as by standardizing the ways in which the findings from such trials are reported. The CONSORT checklist includes 22 items that should be included in reports describing RCTs, and its accompanying flowchart outlines how patients move through the trial process. The CONSORT statement is published in several languages and has received the endorsement of several prominent medical journals, including *The Lancet, Annals of Internal Medicine*, and the *Journal of the American Medical Association (JAMA)*. As of 2002, CONSORT was being used by about 500 journals, most leading editorial groups, and many granting agencies (Moher, 2002). Wider dissemination of the CONSORT guidelines within the CAM community (Moher, 2002) should improve the quality of reports of CAM-related RCTs in the future. A related document, the QUOROM statement, provides specific guidelines for the reporting of meta-analyses of RCTs, as well as a checklist and flow diagram to promote standardization and the inclusion of critical components. The CONSORT and QUOROM checklists and diagrams are available at http://www. con-sort-statement.org.

Similarly, STRICTA provides a set of guidelines based on the CONSORT statement and is meant to serve as an acupuncture-oriented supplement to the CONSORT guidelines. An international group of acupuncture practitioners and researchers established STRICTA guideliness to promote accurate and adequate reporting of acupuncture trials; editors of several journals have also contributed to the drafting of these guidelines. Participating journals publish the STRICTA guidelines and ask their prospective authors to adhere to the standards (MacPherson et al., 2001).

Although CAM therapies are often criticized for being used despite a lack of evidence, hundreds of systematic reviews have, in fact, evaluated specific CAM therapies; of these, some have been well conducted and have shown that the CAM therapy offers a clear benefit. Much more research is required however to demonstrate clearly whether other commonly used therapies are effective. Unfortunately, funding for CAM trials and systematic reviews is limited and generally must come from public resources. Private industry rarely funds research on CAM because the ability to patent natural products or CAM therapies is low. The evidence base for conventional medicine is also not complete, and as discussed above with respect to the study of Ezzo et al. (2001), systematic reviews demonstrate that only 22.5 percent of conventional medicine interventions have a clearly positive effect. Comparisons of quality of systematic reviews of CAM and conventional medicine therapies have shown that they share similar weaknesses (Moher et al., 2002). One of the most important omissions in systematic reviews was a lack of consistent reporting about the methods used to evaluate and assess the quality of the primary studies reviewed (Moher et al., 2002).

Twenty years ago very few RCTs of CAM therapies had been conducted, and the systematic review methodology was in its infancy. In the past twenty years, however, remarkable progress has been made in terms of the number of trials of CAM therapies conducted, improvements in trial quality, the development of systematic review methods for evaluating such trials, and the development of the infrastructure of the Cochrane Collaboration to support such rigorous evaluations. Although much work remains to be done, a great deal has been accomplished in a short time, from improvements to the indexing terms used and the creation of databases to the establishment of reporting guidelines and quality measurements.

As a result of these efforts, true evidence-based CAM is becoming a reality. With continued financial and institutional support, the success of this enterprise will continue into the future. Efforts to provide evidence-based CAM would be greatly facilitated by a system(s) that could be used to identify, within each agency of the federal government, completed and ongoing research on CAM therapies. Such a system would enable investigators to more quickly and accurately review what is known about various areas of CAM. The clinical trial registry sponsored by NIH and the Food and Drug Administration provides useful information on clinical trials; however, other research activities on CAM are not included in this registry. Therefore, **the committee recommends that the federal government develop systems that can be used to identify CAM research and expenditures at the**

National Institutes of Health, the Centers for Disease Control and Prevention, the Health Resources Service Administration, Medicare, Medicaid, the U.S. Department of Agriculture, the U.S. Department of Defense, the U.S. Department of Veterans Affairs, and other federal agencies as appropriate.

The following section describes some of the gaps in evidence for CAM therapies and explores options that can be used to fill those gaps.

GAPS IN EVIDENCE

The scientific evidence that is developing in CAM research, reviewed earlier in this chapter, is primarily based on findings from clinical research on CAM treatments. This clinical research, which is itself still in a nascent phase and which is sometimes flawed, represents just one facet of the research that is needed. There are very large gaps in basic research on the underlying mechanisms through which CAM treatments affect outcomes, clinical research that compares CAM interventions with the interventions used in conventional medicine, and cost-effectiveness and health care utilization studies. Furthermore, as discussed in Chapter 4, advances in CAM are dependent on the ability to address complex methodological challenges created by the unique characteristics of CAM therapies.

Clinical Research

Although most research on CAM is clinical, there is a paucity of clinical research in which CAM interventions are compared with each other or with conventional medicine interventions. As discussed in Chapter 4, one of the obstacles to comparing CAM treatments with conventional medicine treatments is that CAM treatments often consider outcomes that are not ordinarily considered by conventional medicine research, such as "being centered" or "connectedness to the CAM provider or family members." Conversely, conventional medicine studies often consider outcomes such as functional status and disease-specific outcomes that may not be used in studies of CAM therapies. Each type of medicine—conventional medicine and CAM—should make efforts to include the outcomes of the other type to facilitate valid comparisons between CAM and conventional medicine treatments. For example, measures of mood, quality of life, and preferences for outcome states that are used in clinical studies of conventional medicine therapies could be included in studies of CAM therapies. Measures of the outcomes that are often of interest to CAM patients and providers need to be developed that can then be used in conventional medicine research as well as CAM research. Collaboration between CAM researchers and social and behavioral scientists skilled in measurement development could be fruitful in this regard.

Basic Science

A great opportunity for scientific discovery in the basic science of CAM treatments is at hand. Of the basic research that has been done, botanicals have probably received the greatest amount of attention, in the form of studies of individual botanicals, botanical-drug interactions, and the identification of new drugs. NCCAM, like other institutes, centers, and offices of NIH, is giving a high priority to studies to determine the active ingredients, dosing, pharmacology, stability, and bioavailability of CAM therapies (NCCAM, 2004). Some of the formative research in this area has produced findings on the lack of identification of isoflavonone formononetin in a variety of black cohosh (*Cimicifuga racemosa*) populations. Isoflavonone formononetin is believed to be important in the reduction of menopausal vasomotor symptoms, and the findings of research of black cohosh given to menopausal women indicate that estrogen activity is due to compounds other than formononetin (Kennelly et al., 2002). Licorice root (*Glycrrhiza glabra)* induces apoptosis, G2/M cell cycle arrest, and Bcl-2 phosphorylation in tumor cell lines (Rafi et al., 2002), and pharmacokinetic studies of purified soy isoflavones show that high doses are rapidly eliminated by healthy males resulting in minimal toxicity (Busby et al., 2002). These are only a handful of the high-quality investigations on the basic science of medicinal plants that have been reported, while many others have been completed or are ongoing.

The area of mind-body medicine also offers exciting opportunities for basic research. Advances in technology enable research, for example, on the effects of mind-body techniques such as the effects of meditation on the brain, the endocrine system, and the immune system. New imaging techniques make it possible to study the phenomenon of acupuncture analgesia and placebo effects. For example, ter Riet et al. (1998) conducted a systematic review of six studies on the mechanism of placebo analgesia in humans and concluded that the studies provide evidence that a placebo analgesia effect exists. Pollo et al. (2001) examined whether expectations about treatment influence analgesic effects. They found that "different verbal instructions about certain and uncertain expectations of analgesia produce different placebo analgesic effects, which in turn trigger a dramatic change of behavior leading to a significant reduction of opioid intake". These are but a few of many examples of areas of inquiry that hold great promise for understanding basic mechanisms of action relevant to the practice of CAM.

Cost-Effectiveness Studies

Although a number of clinical studies are examining the efficacies of CAM treatments, very little research has tracked the costs associated with the treatment outcomes. Research on the cost-effectiveness of CAM therapies is hindered by a lack of consistency of treatments, a lack of standardized coding, and defects in clinical trials (pertinent to both conventional medicine and CAM treatment trials). These defects include the fact that the clinical trials are underpowered, a lack of an adequate description of subject recruitment, the use of suboptimal controls, and the use of single-center trials, which threatens generalizability and power.

Cross-Disciplinary Research

Research on CAM treatments benefits from the contributions of more than one discipline. In addition to providers who have specialized knowledge of CAM treatments and methodologists who can address the challenges inherent in CAM research design, CAM research can benefit by the inclusion of scientists with backgrounds in fields such as psychology, sociology, anthropology, economics, genetics, pharmacology, neuroscience, health services research, and health policy. These individuas can address the multiplicity of factors that influence those who use CAM treatments and the outcomes of those treatments.

Engaging experts from multiple fields in the investigation of CAM therapies provides an excellent opportunity to conduct transdisciplinary research. "*Transdisciplinary research* involves broadly constituted teams of researchers that work across disciplines in the development of the research questions to be addressed" (IOM, 2003b). Transdiciplinary research on CAM therapies could involve teams composed of a rheumatologist, immunologist, neuroscientist, epidemiologist, biostatistician, traditional Chinese medicine practitioner, and physician who is trained in conventional medicine and CAM and is investigating chronic pain disorders such as osteoarthritis.

Research Investigators

Established scientists are drawn to a new field by interesting questions, especially when such questions can be approached by using the scientists' knowledge and skills and by the availability of resources. Relatively few established scientists are engaged in CAM research, however, and certain areas of CAM are ripe for research. Mind-body medicine provides a good example. Mind-body medicine concerns the effects of the brain on biophysiological processes and clinical outcomes. Clinical researchers and basic scientists who share interest in these questions have traditionally pursued their interests separately and have published their findings in different journals. However, the public's growing interest in practices such as meditation as a way of reducing the risk for and recovery from illness is motivating a more clinical orientation by basic scientists and a more basic science orientation by clinical researchers.

Advances in the cognitive and affective neurosciences and technical advances in imaging techniques are fueling the convergence of clinical science and basic science. A study by Davidson et al. (2003) provides a good example of this convergence. These investigators conducted an RCT of the effects of a meditation-based clinical training program on brain and immune function. At the conclusion of the training, subjects in both groups were vaccinated with influenza vaccine. Meditators showed a significant increase in left-sided anterior activation compared with that for the nonmeditators, and they also had a significant increase in antibody titers compared with the titers in the nonmeditators.

Scientists in other areas should be made aware of the exciting questions about CAM that remain to be answered. Such interest can be fanned in a variety of ways, including conferences focused on particular CAM modalities that invite science-oriented CAM practitioners and scientists from other areas to participate. Invitations to scientists to apply their knowledge and skill to CAM research questions will be more attractive if they include certain kinds of collaborations. Both basic research and clinical research in CAM involve subject matter that is likely to be beyond the conventional scientist's knowledge base and scientists new to CAM will often need to be partnered with individuals who are expert in the focal CAM modality. Furthermore, investigation of a number of CAM modalities, such as traditional Chinese medicine, by conventional scientific techniques is scientifically problematic and requires the collaboration of methodologists who can create appropriate and effective research designs (see Chapter 4).

The development of a workforce to conduct research on CAM will proceed more rapidly if critical masses of investigators can be created in various locations. Furthermore, CAM research should thrive in an interdisciplinary environment. Centers that bring together scientists from diverse disciplines can help create these interdisciplinary groups of scientists focused on particular aspects of CAM. The cross-collaborations and synergy that characterize a strong center will contribute to the more rapid growth of a cadre of scientists who will be able to advance the research in CAM.

As discussed in Chapter 1, one of the goals of the Academic Health Centers for Integrative Medicine is to "help transform medicine and health care through rigorous scientific studies" (see Appendix B for a list of centers). One such center at the University of Maryland has grown out of a partnership of funding from private foundations with university support and resources. This combination allowed the start of pilot research projects that could generate preliminary data that were used to make successful applications to NIH for grants for CAM research including a center grant. The University of Maryland model (which started in 1991) has relied on a collaborative team approach whereby clinicians experienced in CAM modalities work with specialists in rheumatology and pain (the particular focus of the center) as well as seasoned methodologists and statisticians to design trials that are sensitive to the unique practice of the CAM modality while meeting the highest methodological standards. The center grant funding has been crucial in establishing various infrastructural cores. For example, the first core, the database and evaluation core, locates the existing literature in the field, synthesizes the data, and conducts systematic reviews to aid in formulating appropriate research hypotheses and designing appropriate studies. Until recently this task was greatly hindered by the fact that CAM journals were not listed in MEDLINE, and literature search strategies such as those that use keywords were inadequate. However, this situation has changed, and many of the difficulties have improved.

A second core of the Maryland center is administrative and provides oversight and management for all stages of the research process. A statistical, epidemiological, and data management core, the third core, provides consultation on all aspects of study design, data collection, and statistical analysis. Studies funded by the center grant have completed the Phase II level of development, which has led to large, fully developed Phase III clinical trials, in addition to allowing transitional research from basic science studies through clinical trials. Furthermore, a program of development and feasibility studies and a training and education program have built on the concept of a collaborative model, encouraging innovative lines of investigation and the nurturing of new investigators in the field. These programs have allowed the center to bring together experienced investigators from a broad range of medical disciplines to work with the center team on pilot research studies, and it has also mentored junior faculty and postdoctoral fellows as they develop lines of inquiry and embark on independent careers in the field.

The field of CAM also needs a cadre of new junior researchers. Models of training programs in basic and clinical research for conventional medicine can be found in major U.S. health sciences campuses. The challenge is to induce such programs to include training in clinical research for CAM. One approach is to build upon existing research training programs by adding specific CAM content for the trainees in CAM. This could be done through postdoctoral training programs that are designed for basic and clinical research in conventional medicine. This is an efficient way to develop CAM researchers during the period when not enough CAM researchers are available to serve as faculty for a complete program. A second approach is to provide supplemental grants to existing grants that will fund a junior researcher to conduct CAM research and benefit from mentoring by the principal investigator of the existing grant. NIH has used this approach to help increase the numbers of researchers from under-represented minorities. A third approach is to award individual career development grants that allow the junior researcher of CAM to be trained by established researchers from around the country. A fourth approach is to provide intensive workshops at a central location followed by mentoring and technical support for the participants when they return to their home institutions.

All the approaches described above involve programs for people with conventional M.D. or Ph.D. training. Chapter 8 discusses the training of CAM practitioners to conduct research. The next section explores a frame-work for research and the translation of validated therapies into practice.

A RESEARCH FRAMEWORK

During its deliberations and analyses, the committee concluded that research on CAM is inextricably linked to the practice of CAM therapies for many reasons, an important one of which is that CAM therapies are already in widespread use today and it is reasonable to attempt to evaluate the outcomes of that use. Another is that in the practice setting one can focus on research that answers questions about how therapies function in the real world where patients vary, often have multiple problems, and are using multiple therapies. Such a focus not only generates research that addresses real-world practice issues but also facilitates the adoption of practice changes on the basis of those research results (Green and Dovey, 2001; Nutting et al., 1999). Therefore, the committee believes that it is equally important both to continue to conduct research aimed at determin-ing efficacy and uncovering mechanisms of action *and* to engage in research aimed at investigating what is occurring in practice. Furthermore, the gath-ering and analysis of accurate information about CAM (and conventional medicine) practices and their use are crucial to measuring and understand-ing outcomes of care.

Chapter 2 of this report discussed what is known about the use of CAM by the American public. That chapter also described how little infor-mation is available about

- CAM use by specific populations;
- how the American public gathers and evaluates information and makes decisions about accessing CAM therapies;
  - what motivates patients to use CAM;
  - adherence to CAM treatment or self-treatment with CAM;

- outcomes, including adverse events, of single CAM therapies, multiple CAM therapies, and CAM therapies in combination with conventional therapies; and
- the extent to which CAM use is a trigger for positive behavioral change.

This chapter discusses what is known about the efficacy and effectiveness of CAM therapies and the need for additional basic science, cost-effectiveness, and cross-disciplinary research in CAM. To address these gaps, the committee has developed the research model illustrated in Figure 5-3. Four major components of this model are national surveys (both periodic and longitudinal surveys), a sentinel surveillance system, practice-based research networks (PBRNs), and CAM research centers.

National Surveys

The first component of the research model illustrated in Figure 5-3 is a set of interactive surveys. Data from these surveys are needed to capture CAM use by the American public in a timely manner for several distinct, but interrelated purposes. First, there is a need for periodic (e.g., every 5 years), large, comprehensive surveys assessing the prevalence, patterns, perceptions, and costs of CAM therapy use by a representative national survey of adults living in the United States. This will provide data on national trends on CAM use that will enable comparisons over time by class of patient, e.g., by ethnicity, gender, area of the country, insurance status, and the general rate of use of CAM. In designing such surveys, oversampling of various ethnic minority populations is necessary to ensure the collection of high-quality data that document the differences in the patterns of CAM use by both preference and level of access to all types of health care services among minority (and majority) populations.

Second, questions related to CAM should be included on annual and semiannual federally funded surveys focusing on the health care of the American public. The recently completed study by the National Center for Health Statistics is an excellent example of the type of survey needed (Barnes et al., 2004). It is also important to establish a set of common questions that can be rotated (because of time constraints) to enable the more frequent tracking of a core set of key variables (e.g., prevalence of CAM use, major disease categories treated by CAM, average numbers of visits by CAM users, and out-of-pocket expenditures).

Third, questions related to CAM should be included on ongoing, longitudinal, cohort studies to enable documentation of the patterns of CAM use over time and their relationship (or lack thereof) to health outcomes. Longitudinal cohort studies have produced data that result in major benefits to

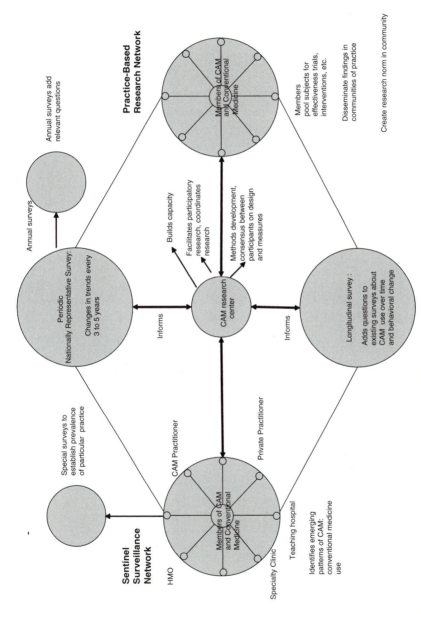

FIGURE 5-3 A model for CAM research and translation.

the public's health. For example, data from the Multiple Risk Factor Intervention Trial and the Framingham Heart Study revealed the importance of preventing "development of unfavorable levels of blood cholesterol and blood pressure, cigarette smoking, diabetes, and unfavorable body weight" as crucial to preventing clinical coronary heart disease (Greenland et al., 2003).

The ideal situation would be the inclusion of CAM-related questions in such studies as the National Health and Nutrition Examination Survey (NHANES) study, the Behavioral Risk Factor Surveillance Survey, the Framingham Heart Study, or the Nurses' Health Study. This would enable investigators to examine the impact of CAM use over time on the health of individuals as well as the members of a particular cohort.

Finally, surveys that are explicitly intended to capture the real and the perceived adverse events associated with CAM use should be established. The results of such surveys could be used to identify high-priority research topics.

The information produced by the types of surveys described above is crucial to understanding the use of CAM therapies in the United States and prioritization of the CAM-related research portfolio. These surveys form a key component of the model illustrated in Figure 5-3. Although they are extremely valuable, large national surveys are unable to monitor emergent patterns of CAM use, the specifics of CAM use, and particular combinations of CAM use for particular purposes. Other types of data need to be collected to explore such things as how CAM use is associated with behavioral change or is related to risk and health-protective or health-promotive behaviors. Another key component of that model, the sentinel surveillance system, plays an important role in answering these types of questions by providing timely information about treatment trends that demand research and is described below.

Sentinel Surveillance System

Surveillance is defined as "ongoing systematic collection, analysis and interpretation of data and the distribution to those who need to know" (Thacker and Berkelman, 1988). Surveillance has many uses when it is well designed and implemented and can be used to

- obtain quantitative estimates of the magnitude of a health problem;
- portray the natural history of disease;
- detect epidemics;
- document the distribution and spread of a health event;
- facilitate epidemiological and laboratory research;

- test a hypothesis;
- evaluate control and prevention measures;
- monitor changes in the prevalence of infectious agents;
- monitor isolation activities;
- monitor behavioral change-associated risk or prevention of illness;
- monitor public receptiveness to marketing and public health messages—i.e., information;
- detect changes in health care practices; and
- plan (Thacker, 1992).

Groseclose and colleagues (2000) classify surveillance systems as either *passive* or *active*. Passive surveillance reporting systems can provide incomplete information because they depend on the voluntary reporting of data. *Active* surveillance systems, on the other hand, solicit data from selected sites for specific purposes, for example, the use of particular antibiotics for a condition like otitis media. A *sentinel surveillance system* can be either active or passive and is composed of selected sites that report information that may be generalizable to the population as a whole (Birkhead and Maylahn, 2000). Sentinel sites (both CAM and conventional medicine) might include practitioners, hospitals, specialty clinics, clinics that serve specific population subgroups, health maintenance organizations, and teaching hospitals that have agreed to report information. Member sites might serve either a common population defined by a particular set of health problems or a particular population (by age, ethnicity, location, etc.).

The value of sentinel surveillance systems can be seen in the public health system, in which they "have been particularly helpful in monitoring specific infections or designated classes of infections" (IOM, 2003a). The Emerging Infections Program, a surveillance system collaboration among the Centers for Disease Control and Prevention, state public health departments, and other public health partners, conducts surveillance for unexplained deaths and severe illnesses to "identify diseases and infectious agents, known and unknown, that can lead to severe illness or death" (IOM, 2003a).

For CAM, a sentinel surveillance system is important to monitoring changes in the American public's use of CAM alone or in combination with conventional medicine, thereby highlighting high-priority areas for practice-based research.

The third major component of the model described in Figure 5-3 is practice-based research networks. The following discussion describes the value and importance of such networks both to effectiveness research and to the translation of validated therapies into practice.

Practice-Based Research Networks

Nutting (1996) writes, "In the primary care setting, patients present with multiple problems: some are diseases, others are illnesses that may become diseases, and many are neither, yet all are important and can measurably decrease function and quality of life." Although, Nutting was referring to conventional primary care, the description also holds for patients who seek CAM therapies or both CAM and conventional. He also describes the need to determine practice-relevant research questions, to develop research that draws on the strengths and experiences of practitioners, and to ensure that rigorous and multiple research methods are used for study, concluding that PBRNs are best able to incorporate these and other necessary elements. Nutting is not alone in his belief that PBRNs are vital to effective primary care. Other individuals and organizations also support the development of PBRNs to increase the research and evidence base in primary care (Fenton et al., 2001; Genel and Dobs, 2003; Green and Dovey, 2001; IOM, 1996; Lindbloom et al., 2004).

PBRNs are defined as "a group of ambulatory practices devoted principally to the primary care of patients, affiliated with each other (and often with an academic or professional organization) in order to investigate questions related to community-based practice" (AHRQ, 2001). The 1996 IOM report *Primary Care: America's Health in a New Era*, states, "The committee sees practice-based research networks as a significant underpinning for studies in primary care, noting not only their attractiveness conceptually but the growing recognition of their value" (IOM, 1996). That report recommend that "the Department of Health and Human Services provide adequate and stable financial support to practice-based primary care research networks."

According to Thomas et al. (2001), PBRNs emerged in the United Kingdom in the 1960s. Several regional networks were begun in the United States during the 1970s with the first national network established in 1981 (Lindbloom et al., 2004). The Federation of Practice Based Networks, established in 1997, advocates and builds capacity for practice-based research and works to facilitate communication and collaboration among networks (FPBRN, 2004).

Thomas and colleagues (2001) suggest that PBRNs are virtual organizations that to succeed need to specify membership criteria, accountability, and authority; address issues of governance; and evaluate activities. They have identified three network leadership types. In the first type, "practitioners develop their own ideas and the network is led by a peer group," thus facilitating participation because the direction is provided by the practitioners involved. The second type uses a top-down approach with "strong institutional links and research projects led by experts." This approach fosters rapid research of high quality. The third type of network is referred to as "whole systems," in which the leadership is multidisciplinary. Network participants form coalitions including both research experts and novices. According to Thomas et al. (2001), the whole systems approach is good for producing cultural change because different enthusiasts in different parts of the health care system become involved.

Griffiths and colleagues (2000) describe different network organizational styles in the following manner:

> . . . some have a hierarchical organisation with a strong centre, often at a university, leading satellite units or network members; others are less hierarchical with coordination and cooperation between satellite units and members as well as with the centre.

Despite differences in design and organization, Nutting et al. (1999) describe four central characteristics of all PBRNs:

1. PBRNs capture health care events that reflect the selection and observer bias that characterize primary care in community-based patient populations.
2. PBRNs provide access to the practice experience and care provided by full-time primary care clinicians.
3. PBRNs focus their activities on practice-relevant research questions, apply appropriate multimethod research designs, and generally avoid the tendency to permit research methods to define the question.
4. Networks strive for the systematic involvement of network clinicians in defining the research questions, participating in the study design, and interpreting study results.

PBRNs conduct studies that use both qualitative and quantitative methods ranging from observational studies to RCTs. For example, using observational data from The Direct Observation of Primary Care Study, Stange et al. (1998) found "that family physicians target preventive services toward patients most in need of them and use illness visits as opportunities for prevention"; a randomized control trial by Fleming et al. "provided the first direct evidence that brief physician intervention was effective in reducing alcohol use and utilization of health care services" (Nutting et al., 1999). Some networks focus on providing epidemiological data; others are concerned with the process of care (Griffiths et al., 2000).

A PBRN can provide information on the content and the practice patterns offered in various types of clinical settings, offer flexibility in collecting and analyzing data from a variety of perspectives (e.g., the practitioner and the patient), provide the opportunity to ask and answer practice-relevant questions, and study CAM treatments in the manner in which they are practiced. Once a PBRN is in place, the additional costs of mounting specific studies can be fairly low, and the level of preparedness engendered by its structure can allow the timely generation of research findings (Zarin et al., 1997). An additional benefit of PBRNs, especially in the area of CAM, which has historically lacked a research infrastructure, is their potential to provide places of learning, provide training in research, and, through direct involvement of practitioners with science, promote a climate of inquiry that both questions and increases the evidence underlying a particular practice.

Furthermore, according to Genel and Dobs (2003), PBRNs can facilitate the translation of research findings into practice. They assert that PBRNs address two of the greatest difficulties in translating findings into practice: the lack of communication between academic and practicing physicians and the failure to address practitioner needs in research. Genel and Dobs assert that practitioners must be trained in clinical research and that, as their familiarity with that research grows, they will be enthusiastic about the research effort and will be more likely to implement the research results in their own practices.

CAM Research Centers

The fourth major component of the research model proposed here is a CAM Research Center. Currently, NCCAM funds specialized research centers, each of which focuses on research in one particular area (see Appendix F for a list of these centers). For example, the center at the Oregon Health Sciences University focuses on CAM research in neurological disorders; the center at Columbia University investigates CAM use in aging; the center at the University of California at Los Angeles fosters research evaluating safety and efficacy of botanical dietary supplements; and the center at the University of Illinois at Chicago is studying botanical dietary supplements for women's health.

The CAM research centers envisioned in the committee's research framework differ from these specialized research centers in important ways. First, they are not restricted to one central focus. Rather they would facilitate the activities of the research networks across many topic areas. The centers in Figure 5-3 would propose (or seek input from the network for) specific research questions and protocols. They would help coordinate the design and implementation of these investigations; coordinate refinement of protocols and priorities over time; and supervise the analyses of data generated from these studies. Unlike NCCAM centers as currently structured and funded, these new centers require a much broader spectrum of expertise from both the conventional and CAM research and clinical communities because they would not be focused on one modality or one clinical problem. These centers must have the capacity to work with the networks to identify important questions and to design studies that are hypothesis generating and hypothesis testing.

The proposed centers coordinate data collection and analysis—bringing in information gleaned through longitudinal and periodic studies as well as data collected by the surveillance sites—and provide research and other training to network and surveillance participants as needed. In some instances, it is likely that they will serve in the more traditional role of a coordinating site for multisite observational or controlled trials, but this is not the main or sole purpose of their creation.

The committee believes strongly that the center team should be transdisciplinary, at a minimum composed of methodologists, social and behavioral scientists, and experienced integrative medicine practitioners. As the network evolves it is anticipated that individuals from other disciplines would join the coordinating team. This team should be committed to a participatory research process and the cannons of conducting good science.

These four major components, national surveys, a sentinel surveillance system, practice-based research networks, and CAM research centers, form the core of the research, reporting, and translation model developed by the committee and illustrated in Figure 5-3.

A Model for CAM Research and Surveillance

In the model for CAM research and surveillance shown in Figure 5-3 the left-hand hub represents the sentinel surveillance function. Sentinel surveillance sites would be responsible for the systematic collection and reporting of data on common and emerging patterns of CAM use as well as the use of both CAM and conventional medicine. Such information could be used to identify treatment trends that demand research. A sentinel surveillance approach to the collection of data on the use of CAM would complement the periodic population-based survey approach because data would be collected in an ongoing fashion in contexts subject to real-world contingencies and for a variety of different populations. The sentinel surveillance systems formed in different parts of the country would also provide data that allow the monitoring and analysis of regional and national trends in CAM use.

Another advantage of sentinel surveillance systems relates to the translation of research results into practice. That is, such systems allow the real-time monitoring of the impact of the information about various CAM treatments disseminated to the public and practitioners by asking such questions as How does information influence practice? and How does treatment affect behaviorial change? The information collected by the sentinel sites could then be reported to the CAM research center (center of

Figure 5-3), where it would be reviewed to determine whether emerging patterns that would be useful to study may exist.

The right-hand hub of Figure 5-3 is the PBRN. Network participants would be recruited from many disciplines and would include both CAM and conventional medicine practitioners. It is anticipated that this network will conduct practice-based participatory research. Practitioners involved in the PBRN will learn research study designs through their preparation for and participation in network search activities. Additionally, these practitioners will be in a position to guide the development of new instruments and outcome measures of relevance to the community.

In the model illustrated in Figure 5-3, the CAM research center would work with the PBRN to develop a consensus on how best to test the effectiveness and safety of treatments and bundles of behavior associated with treatment approaches. Together, the center and the network would

- Select target conditions to be evaluated
- Develop a protocol designed to capture
  —Health care practices engaged in by patients as self-care
  —Health care administered or prescribed by practitioners
  —Interactions between self-care and practitioner care and between conventional medical care and CAM care
  —Notable lifestyle changes that may effect health status, e.g., interactions between medication use and special diets the population has adopted
  —Exposure of the population to marketing and public health messages
- Identify sites attending to patients (by both CAM and conventional medicine) with the targeted conditions
- Organize the data collection on the basis of an agreed-upon sampling procedure
- Develop an effectiveness study or intervention activity linked to the surveillance data

It is the committee's belief that the model for research and translation illustrated and described above would provide a coordinated mechanism directed at answering the myriad questions about CAM use, such as Who is using CAM and why are they doing so? and Are CAM therapies safe, effective, and cost-effective? The committee strongly urges NIH and other public agencies to provide the support necessary to develop and implement such a model.

CONCLUSIONS AND RECOMMENDATIONS

Both Chapter 2 and this chapter have presented information on what is known about CAM and where the gaps in knowledge exist. Chapter 2 presented the committee's recommendations on ways to address the gaps in knowledge discussed in that chapter. These gaps in knowledge are reviewed below:

• The information available about the motivations for CAM use indicates that pursuit of wellness is a major impetus; however, the extent to which CAM use is a trigger for positive behavioral change is unknown and constitutes an important research issue.

• Existing surveys provide little information about how the use of CAM therapies is initiated; that is, are they self-initiated, provider initiated, provider administered, or self-administered?

• There are virtually no data on adherence to CAM treatment or self-treatment with CAM. This information is crucial to assessments of the real-world effectiveness and safety of CAM therapies and their use.

• Longitudinal studies are needed to clarify people's trajectories of CAM use and those factors that influence upward and downward slopes in use.

• There is little research on how the public obtains information about CAM therapies: what types of information are deemed credible, marginal, and spurious; how does the public understand the information in terms of risks and benefits; how do such perceptions inform decision making; and what do members of the public expect their providers to tell them?

This chapter has discussed the emerging evidence about CAM therapies, including sources of information (MEDLINE, The Cochrane Library); summarized the systematic reviews that have been conducted; examined the need for high-quality studies; and explored the gaps in evidence. The gaps discussed include the paucity of clinical research in which CAM interventions are compared with each other and with conventional medicine therapies, the need for expanded basic research to include areas other than botanicals, the lack of cost-effectiveness research, the need for cross-disciplinary and transdisciplinary research, and the importance of drawing established scientists to the field of CAM research. The committee has proposed a research framework to address these gaps as well as conduct the kinds of research recommended in Chapter 2. This framework includes a sentinel surveillance system, PBRNs, and CAM research centers that can incorporate information from national surveys (both periodic and longitudinal) and facilitate the work of the PBRNs.

The committee believes that a research model such as the one described in this chapter, if it is adequately funded and implemented, will help provide additional understanding of the vast and varied field of CAM. As part of the following recommendation, the committee specifies the need for oversampling of racial and ethnic minorities in surveys. Many racial and ethnic minorities constitute a comparatively small proportion of the total U.S. population or are concentrated in a small number of geographic areas. In both situations, the number of individuals in a specific racial or ethnic group who will be selected in a nationwide random sample is typically too small to provide the basis for statistically reliable estimates for that population. Therefore, the only way to obtain meaningful results for such minority groups and to allow comparisons with the majority non-Hispanic white population is to oversample these groups, that is, to select the sample in a fashion that ensures that the proportion of individuals from these minority groups in the sample is larger than their proportion in the overall U.S. population.

The committee recommends that the National Institutes of Health and other public agencies provide the support necessary to
- **develop and implement a sentinel surveillance system, practice-based research networks, and CAM research centers to facilitate the work of the networks;**
- **include CAM-relevant questions in federally funded health care surveys (e.g., the National Health Interview Survey) and in ongoing longitudinal cohort studies (e.g., the Nurses' Health Study and the Framingham Heart Study); and**
- **implement periodic comprehensive, representative, national surveys to assess the changes in the prevalence, patterns, perceptions, and costs of therapy use (both CAM and conventional medicine), with oversampling of ethnic minorities.**

REFERENCES

AHRQ (Agency for Healthcare Research and Quality). 2001. *Primary Care Practice-Based Research Networks*. [Online]. Available: http://www.ahrq.gov/research/pbrnfact.htm [accessed June 16, 2004].

Allen C, Clark M. 2003. International Activity Within Collaborative Review Groups. In: *11th Cochrane Colloquium: Evidence, Healthcare and Culture*. Oxford, UK: U.K. Cochrane Center. P. 44.

Atallah AN, Hofmeyr GJ, Duley L. Calcium supplementation during pregnancy for preventing hypertensive disorders and related problems. *Cochrane Database Syst Rev* 2004; (1).

Barnes PM, Powell-Griner E, McFann K, Nahin RL. 2004. Complementary and alternative medicine use among adults: United States, 2002. *Vital Health Stat* 343:1–19 (advance data).

Bausell RB, Lee WL, Li YF, Soeken KS, Berman BM. 2004. Larger effect sizes were associated with higher quality ratings in complementary and alternative medicine randomized controlled trials. *J Clin Epidemiol* 57(5):438–446.

Beckles Willson N, Elliott TM, Everard ML. Omega-3 fatty acids (from fish oils) for cystic fibrosis. *Cochrane Database Syst Rev* 2004; (1).

Birkhead GS, Maylahn CM. 2000. *State and Local Public Health Surveillance in Principles and Practice of Public Health Surveillance.* Teutsch SM, Churchill RE, eds. New York: Oxford University Press. Pp. 253–287.

Brosseau L, Yonge KA, Robinson V, Marchand S, Judd M, Wells G, Tugwell P. Transcutaneous electrical nerve stimulation (TENS) for the treatment of rheumatoid arthritis in the hand. *Cochrane Database Syst Rev* 2004; (1).

Busby MG, Jeffcoat AR, Bloedon LT, Koch MA, Black T, Dix KJ, Heizer WD, Thomas BF, Hill JM, Crowell JA, Zeisel SH. 2002. Clinical characteristics and pharmacokinetics of purified soy isoflavones: Single-dose administration to healthy men. *Am J Clin Nutr* 75(1):126–136.

Caraballoso M, Sacristan M, Serra C, Bonfill X. 2003. Drugs for preventing lung cancer in healthy people. *Cochrane Database Syst Rev* 2:CD002141.

Caraballoso M, Sacristan M, Serra C, Bonfill X. Drugs for preventing lung cancer in healthy people. *Cochrane Database Syst Rev* 2004; (1).

D'Souza RM, D'Souza R. Vitamin A for treating measles in children. *Cochrane Database Syst Rev* 2004; (1).

Darlow B, Austin N. Selenium supplementation to prevent short-term morbidity in preterm neonates. *Cochrane Database Syst Rev* 2004; (4).

Darlow BA, Graham PJ. Vitamin A supplementation for preventing morbidity and mortality in very low birthweight infants. *Cochrane Database Syst Rev* 2004; (4).

Davidson RJ, Kabat-Zinn J, Schumacher J, Rosenkranz M, Muller D, Santorelli SF, Urbanowski F, Harrington A, Bonus K, Sheridan JF. 2003. Alterations in brain and immune function produced by mindfulness meditation. *Psychosom Med* 65(4):564–570.

Dickersin K, Manheimer E. 1998. The Cochrane Collaboration: Evaluation of health care and services using systematic reviews of the results of randomized controlled trials. *Clin Obstet Gynecol* 41(2):315–331.

Dickersin K, Scherer R, Lefebvre C. 1994. Identifying relevant studies for systematic reviews. *BMJ* 309(6964):1286–1291.

Douglas RM, Chalker EB, Treacy B. Vitamin C for preventing and treating the common cold. *Cochrane Database Syst Rev* 2004; (1).

Egger M, Juni P, Bartlett C, Holenstein F, Sterne J. 2003. How important are comprehensive literature searches and the assessment of trial quality in systematic reviews? Empirical study. *Health Technol Assess* 7(1):1–76.

Eisenberg DM, Davis RB, Ettner SL, Appel S, Wilkey S, Van Rompay M, Kessler RC. 1998. Trends in alternative medicine use in the United States, 1990-1997: Results of a follow-up national survey. *JAMA* 280(18):1569–1575.

Evans JR. Antioxidant vitamin and mineral supplements for age-related macular degeneration. *Cochrane Database Syst Rev* 2004; (1).

Ezzo J, Bausell B, Moerman DE, Berman B, Hadhazy V. 2001. Reviewing the reviews. How strong is the evidence? How clear are the conclusions? *Int J Technol Assess Health Care* 17(4):457–466.

Farmer A, Montori V, Dinneen S, Clar C. Fish oil in people with type 2 diabetes mellitus. *Cochrane Database Syst Rev* 2004; (1).

Fenton E, Harvey J, Griffiths F, Wild A, Sturt J. 2001. Reflections from organization science on the development of primary health care research networks. *Fam Pract* 18(5):540–544.

FPBRN (Federation of Practice Based Research Networks). 2004. *Federation of Practice Based Research Networks Homepage.* [Online]. Available: http://www.aafp.org/x19544.xml [accessed April 14, 2004].

Furlan AD, Brosseau L, Imamura M, Irvin E. Massage for low back pain. *Cochrane Database Syst Rev* 2004; (1).

Friedman R, Sobel D, Myers P, Caudill M, Benson H. 1995. Behavioral medicine, clinical health psychology, and cost offset. *Health Psychol* 14(6):509–518.

Genel M, Dobs A. 2003. Translating clinical research into practice: Practice-based research networks—a promising solution. *J Investig Med* 51(2):64–71.

Green LA, Dovey SM. 2001. Practice based primary care research networks. They work and are ready for full development and support. *BMJ* 322(7286):567–568.

Greenland P, Knoll MD, Stamler J, Neaton JD, Dyer AR, Garside EB, Wilson PW. 2003. Major risk factors as antecedents of fatal and nonfatal coronary heart disease events. *JAMA* 290:891–897.

Griffiths F, Wild A, Harvey J, Fenton E. 2000. The productivity of primary care research networks. *Br J Gen Pract* 50(460):913–915.

Grol R, Grimshaw J. 2003. From best evidence to best practice: Effective implementation of change in patients' care. *Lancet* 362(9391):1225–1230.

Groseclose SL, Sullivan KM, Gibbs NP, Knowles CM. 2000. Management of the Surveillance Information System and Quality Control of Data. In: Teutsch SM, Churchill RE, eds. *Principles and Practice of Public Health Surveillance.* New York: Oxford University Press. Pp. 95–112.

Health Forum/American Hospital Association. 2003. *2003 Complementary and Alternative Medicine Survey.* [Online]. Available: http://www.hospitalconnect.com/aha/resource_center/statistics/Complementary%20and%20Alternative%20Medicine%20Survey.html [accessed June 16, 2004].

Herxheimer A, Petrie KJ. Melatonin for preventing and treating jet lag. *Cochrane Database Syst Rev* 2004; (1).

Homik J, Suarez-Almazor ME, Shea B, Cranney A, Wells G, Tugwell P. Calcium and vitamin D for corticosteroid-induced osteoporosis. *Cochrane Database Syst Rev* 2004; (1).

Howlett A, Ohlsson A. Inositol for respiratory distress syndrome in preterm infants. *Cochrane Database Syst Rev* 2004; (1).

Hulme J, Robinson V, DeBie R, Wells G, Judd M, Tugwell P. Electromagnetic fields for the treatment of osteoarthritis. *Cochrane Database Syst Rev* 2004; (1).

Hypericum Depression Trial Study Group. 2002. Effect of Hypericum perforatum (St John's wort) in major depressive disorder: A randomized controlled trial. *JAMA* 287(14):1807–1814.

IOM (Institute of Medicine). 1996. *Primary Care: America's Health in a New Era.* Washington, DC: National Academy Press.

IOM. 2003a. *The Future of the Public's Health.* Washington, DC: The National Academies Press.

IOM. 2003b. *Who Will Keep the Public Healthy?* Washington, DC: The National Academies Press.

Jadad AR, Moore RA, Carroll D, Jenkinson C, Reynolds DJ, Gavaghan DJ, McQuay HJ. 1996. Assessing the quality of reports of randomized clinical trials: Is blinding necessary? *Control Clin Trials* 17(1):1–12.

Jadad AR, Cook DJ, Jones A, Klassen TP, Tugwell P, Moher M, Moher D. 1998. Methodology and reports of systematic reviews and meta-analyses: A comparison of Cochrane reviews with articles published in paper-based journals. *JAMA* 280(3):278–280.

Jadad AR, Moher M, Browman GP, Booker L, Sigouin C, Fuentes M, Stevens R. 2000. Systematic reviews and meta-analyses on treatment of asthma: Critical evaluation. *BMJ* 320(7234):537–540.

Jepson RG, Mihaljevic L, Craig J. Cranberries for preventing urinary tract infections. *Cochrane Database Syst Rev* 2004; (1).

Juni P, Altman DG, Egger M. 2001. Systematic reviews in health care: Assessing the quality of controlled clinical trials. *BMJ* 323(7303):42–46.

Kennelly EJ, Baggett S, Nuntanakorn P, Ososki AL, Mori SA, Duke J, Coleton M, Kronenberg F. 2002. Analysis of thirteen populations of black cohosh for formononetin. *Phytomedicine* 9(5):461–467.

Lee WL, Bausell RB, Berman BM. 2001. The growth of health-related meta-analyses published from 1980 to 2000. *Evaluation and the Health Professions* 24(3):327–335.

Lindbloom EJ, Ewigman BG, Hickner JM. 2004. Practice-based research networks: The laboratories of primary care research. *Med Care* 42(4 Suppl):III45–III49.

Linde K, Hondras M, Vickers A, ter Riet G, Melchart D. 2001a. Systematic reviews of complementary therapies—An annotated bibliography. Part 3: Homeopathy. *BMC Complemen Altern Med* 1(1):4 (electronic publication).

Linde K, Jonas WB, Melchart D, Willich S. 2001b. The methodological quality of randomized controlled trials of homeopathy, herbal medicines and acupuncture. *Int J Epidemiol* 30(3):526–531.

Linde K, ter Riet G, Hondras M, Vickers A, Saller R, Melchart D. 2001c. Systematic reviews of complementary therapies—An annotated bibliography. Part 2: Herbal medicine. *BMC Complement Altern Med* 1(1):5 (electronic publication).

Linde K, Vickers A, Hondras M, ter Riet G, Thormahlen J, Berman B, Yelchart D. 2001d. Systematic reviews of complementary therapies—An annotated bibliography. Part 1: Acupuncture. *BMC Complement Altern Med* 2001;1(1):3 (electronic publication).

Linde K, Mulrow CD. St John's wort for depression. *Cochrane Database Syst Rev* 2004; (1).

Little CV, Parsons T. Herbal therapy for treating osteoarthritis. *Cochrane Database Syst Rev* 2004; (1).

Lorig KR, Sobel DS, Stewart AL, Brown BW Jr, Bandura A, Ritter P, Gonzalez VM, Laurent DD, Holman HR. 1999. Evidence suggesting that a chronic disease self-management program can improve health status while reducing hospitalization: A randomized trial. *Med Care* 37(1):5–14.

Lumley J, Watson L, Watson M, Bower C. Periconceptional supplementation with folate and/or multivitamins for preventing neural tube defects. *Cochrane Database Syst Rev* 2004; (1).

MacPherson H, White A, Cummings M, Jobst K, Rose K, Niemtzow R. 2001. Standards for reporting interventions in controlled trials of acupuncture: The STRICTA recommendations. *Complement Ther Med* 9(4):246–249.

Mahomed K. Folate supplementation in pregnancy. *Cochrane Database Syst Rev* 2004; (1).

Mahomed K. Iron and folate supplementation in pregnancy. *Cochrane Database Syst Rev* 2004; (1).

Mahomed K. Iron supplementation in pregnancy. *Cochrane Database Syst Rev* 2004; (1).

Manheimer E, Anderson D. 2002. Survey of public information about ongoing clinical trials funded by industry: Evaluation of completeness and accessibility. *BMJ* 325(7363):528–531.

McAlister FA, Laupacis A, Wells GA, Sackett DL. 1999. Users' guides to the medical literature: XIX. Applying clinical trial results B. Guidelines for determining whether a drug is exerting (more than) a class effect. *JAMA* 282(14):1371–1377.

Melchart D, Linde K, Fischer P, Berman B, White A, Vickers A, Allais G. Acupuncture for idiopathic headache. *Cochrane Database Syst Rev* 2004; (1).

Melchart D, Linde K, Fischer P, Kaesmayr J. Echinacea for preventing and treating the common cold. *Cochrane Database Syst Rev* 2004; (1).

Moher D. 2002. The CONSORT guidelines: Improving the quality of research. Consolidated Standards of Reporting Trials. Interview by Bonnie Horrigan. *Altern Ther Health Med* 8(3):103–108.

Moher D, Soeken K, Sampson M, Ben-Porat L, Berman B. 2002. Assessing the quality of reports of systematic reviews in pediatric complementary and alternative medicine. *BMC Pediatr* 2(1):3.

National Institutes of Health. 1998. Acupuncture. NIH Consensus Conference. *JAMA* 280(17):1518–1524.

National Library of Medicine. 2002. *MEDLINE Fact Sheet.* [Online]. Available: http://www. nlm. nih. gov/pubs/factsheets/medline. html [accessed June 16, 2004].

NCCAM (National Center for Complementary and Alternative Medicine). 2004. *Centers for Research on Complementary and Alternative Medicine (CRC) Program FY 2004 Research Priorities.* [Online]. Available: http://nccam. nih. gov/research/priorities/index. htm [accessed June 16, 2004].

Nutting PA. 1996. Practice-based research networks: Building the infrastructure of primary care research. *J Fam Pract* 42(2):199–203.

Nutting PA, Beasley JW, Werner JJ. 1999. Practice-based research networks answer primary care questions. *JAMA* 281(8):686–688.

Ortiz Z, Shea B, Suarez Almazor M, Moher D, Wells G, Tugwell P. Folic acid and folinic acid for reducing side effects in patients receiving methotrexate for rheumatoid arthritis. *Cochrane Database Syst Rev* 2004; (1).

Osiri M, Welch V, Brosseau L, Shea B, McGowan J, Tugwell P, Wells G. Transcutaneous electrical nerve stimulation for knee osteoarthritis. *Cochrane Database Syst Rev* 2004; (1).

Pittler MH, Ernst E. Horse chestnut seed extract for chronic venous insufficiency. *Cochrane Database Syst Rev* 2004; (1).

Pittler MH, Ernst E. Kava extract for treating anxiety. *Cochrane Database Syst Rev* 2004; (1).

Pollo A, Amanzio M, Arslanian A, Casadio C, Maggi G, Benedetti F. 2001. Response expectancies in placebo analgesia and their clinical relevance. *Pain* 93(1):77–84.

Proctor ML, Hing W, Johnson TC, Murphy PA. Spinal manipulation for primary and secondary dysmenorrhoea. *Cochrane Database Syst Rev* 2004; (1).

Proctor ML, Smith CA, Farquhar CM, Stones RW. Transcutaneous electrical nerve stimulation and acupuncture for primary dysmenorrhoea. *Cochrane Database Syst Rev* 2004; (1).

Schulz KF, Chalmers I, Hayes RJ, Altman DG. 1995. Empirical evidence of bias. Dimensions of methodological quality associated with estimates of treatment effects in controlled trials. *JAMA* 273(5):408–412.

Shea B, Wells G, Granney A, Zytaruk N, Robinson V, Griffen L, Hamel C, Ortiz Z, Peterson J, Adachi J, Tugwell P, Guyatt G. Calcium supplementation on bone loss in postmenopausal women. *Cochrane Database Syst Rev* 2004; (1).

Shekelle P, Eccles MP, Grimshaw JM, Woolf SH. 2001. When should clinical guidelines be updated? *BMJ* 323(7305):155–157.

Shiffman RN, Shekelle P, Overhage JM, Slutsky J, Grimshaw J, Deshpande AM. 2003. Standardized reporting of clinical practice guidelines: A proposal from the Conference on Guideline Standardization. *Ann Intern Med* 139(6):493–498.

Silagy CA, Stead LF, Lancaster T. 2001. Use of systematic reviews in clinical practice guidelines: Case study of smoking cessation. *BMJ* 323(7317):833–836.

Stange KC, Zyzanski SJ, Jaen CR, Callahan EJ, Kelly RB, Gillanders WR, Shank JC, Chao J, Medalie JH, Miller WL, Crabtree BF, Flocke SA, Gilchrest VJ, Langa DM, Goodwin MA. 1998. Illuminating the "black box". A description of 4454 patient visits to 138 family physicians. *J Fam Pract* 46:377–389.

Suresh GK, Davis JM, Soll RF. Superoxide dismutase for preventing chronic lung disease in mechanically ventilated preterm infants. *Cochrane Database Syst Rev* 2004; (1).

Tabet N, Birks J, Grimley Evans J. Vitamin E for Alzheimer's disease. *Cochrane Database Syst Rev* 2004; (1).

Tang JL, Wong TW. 1998. The need to evaluate the clinical effectiveness of traditional Chinese medicine. *Hong Kong Med J* 4(2):208–210.

Taylor JA, Weber W, Standish L, Quinn H, Goesling J, McGann M, Calabrese C. 2003. Efficacy and safety of echinacea in treating upper respiratory tract infections in children: A randomized controlled trial. *JAMA* 290(21):2824–2830.

Taylor MJ, Carney S, Geddes J, Goodwin G. Folate for depressive disorders. *Cochrane Database Syst Rev* 2004; (1).

ter Riet G, de Craen AJ, de Boer A, Kessels AG. 1998. Is placebo analgesia mediated by endogenous opioids? A systematic review. *Pain* 76(3):273–275.

Thacker SB. 1992. Les principes et la pratique de la surveillance en santé publique; L'utilization des données en santé publique [The principles and practice of surveillance in public health; The use of data in public health]. *Santé Publique* 1992:43–44.

Thacker SB, Berkelman RL. 1988. Public health surveillance in the United States. *Epidemiol Rev* 10:164–190.

Thomas P, Griffiths F, Kai J, O'Dwyer A. 2001. Networks for research in primary health care. *BMJ* 322(7286):588–590.

Towheed TE, Anastassiades TP, Shea B, Houpt J, Welch V, Hochberg MC. Glucosamine therapy for treating osteoarthritis. *Cochrane Database Syst Rev* 2004; (1).

Vickers A. 1998. Bibliometric analysis of randomized trials in complementary medicine. *Complement Ther Med* 6:185–189.

White AR, Ernst E. 2000. Economic analysis of complementary medicine: A systematic review. *Complement Ther Med* 8(2):111–118.

Wilson ML, Murphy PA. Herbal and dietary therapies for primary and secondary dysmenorrhoea. *Cochrane Database Syst Rev* 2004; (1).

Wilt T, Ishani A, MacDonald R, Rutks I, Stark G. Pygeum africanum for benign prostatic hyperplasia. *Cochrane Database Syst Rev* 2004; (1).

Wilt T, Ishani A, MacDonald R, Stark G, Mulrow C, Lau J. Beta-sitosterols for benign prostatic hyperplasia. *Cochrane Database Syst Rev* 2004; (1).

Wilt T, Ishani A, Stark G, MacDonald R, Mulrow C, Lau J. Serenoa repens for benign prostatic hyperplasia. *Cochrane Database Syst Rev* 2004; (1).

Wilt T, MacDonald R, Ishani A, Rutks I, Stark G. Cernilton for benign prostatic hyperplasia. *Cochrane Database Syst Rev* 2004; (1).

Zarin D, Pincus HA, West J, McIntyre JS. 1997. Practice-based research in psychiatry. *Am J Psychiatry* 154(9):1199–1208.

6

An Ethical Framework for CAM
Research, Practice, and Policy

The statement of task given to the committee necessarily involves consideration of ethical issues. The exploration of the "scientific, policy, and practice questions that arise from the significant and increasing use of complementary and alternative medicine (CAM) therapies by the American public" and "the translation of validated therapies into conventional practice" require that the ethics of medicine be probed in two domains. The first is the individual provision of personal health services; the second is the profession's social advocacy for public health. The statement of task also addresses the development of "models and frameworks" that would be appropriate for the translation of CAM therapies. Ethical models and frameworks for human subjects research as they apply to CAM are an essential part of this development.

VALUE COMMITMENTS THAT INFORM THIS CHAPTER

To accomplish its task, the committee addressed the ethical questions in CAM research, practice, and policy. Yet, even undertaking this task required that some ethical assumptions be made. The committee believes that five major ethical commitments must be embraced. These deserve explicit acknowledgment because they serve as presuppositions or premises of this chapter. The first three are more familiar and will be discussed briefly. The last two receive more expansive treatment because they are less familiar and because they are central to a fair and comprehensive understanding of CAM therapies.

1. A social commitment to public welfare. In terms of medical therapies, a commitment to public welfare is the obligation to generate and provide to health care practitioners, policy makers, and the public access to the best information available on the efficacy of CAM therapies. This is a duty of beneficence (Beauchamp and Childress, 1994; Churchill, 1995).

2. A commitment to protect patients and the public generally from hazardous medical practices and to inform practitioners, policy makers, and the public of select therapeutic modalities that are potentially injurious or deleterious to health. This commitment is closely related to the first one and is often expressed in the bioethics literature as a duty of nonmaleficence, and by physicians as *primum non nocere*—first, do no harm, which comprises the Hippocratic Oath from the sixth century B.C.E. (Beauchamp and Childress, 1994). As will be discussed in this chapter, nonmaleficence in approaching CAM therapies by individual practitioners includes respecting divergent cultural beliefs; creating an emotionally safe environment for the discussion of CAM; and appreciating how CAM may fit into a patient's larger social, familial, or spiritual life (Adams et al., 2002; Cohen, 2003). Nonmaleficence in policy decisions includes such things as devising appropriate research strategies and labeling and advertising policies that protect the public.

3. A respect for patient autonomy (or in social terms, a commitment to consumer choice in health care). Autonomy expresses the interest in allowing and actively enabling individuals to make knowing and voluntary choices in health care, in accord with their own values. Such choices cannot be made without the provision of information regarding benefits and risks that are implied in the first two commitments, so in this way respect for the autonomy of patients (and choice for consumers) is possible only when individuals and social agencies exercise beneficence and nonmaleficence when they are in the position to do so (Beauchamp and Childress, 1994).

4. Recognition of medical pluralism (Callahan, 2002; Kaptchuk and Eisenberg, 2001). Serious consideration of the safety, efficacy, and potential integration of CAM therapies into conventional medicine means acknowledgement of multiple valid modes of healing and a pluralistic foundation for health care. Many CAM practices (such as chiropractic, acupuncture, naturopathy, and homeopathy) are rooted, at least in part, in forms of evidence and logic other than those used in biomedical sciences, often with long traditions and theoretical systems of interpretation divergent from those used in biomedicine. Investigation of CAM practices entails a moral commitment of openness to diverse interpretations of health and healing, a commitment to finding innovative ways of obtaining evidence, and an expansion of the knowledge base relevant and appropriate to medical practice. This commitment to openness also includes reconsideration of

the meaning and the relevance of ethical norms that guide various research and clinical activities, as discussed below.

The recognition of medical pluralism is one way to honor social pluralism, that is, the broad differences in preferences and values expressed through the public's prevalent use of CAM modalities. From a societal perspective, the effort to investigate CAM practices sensitively and analytically means acknowledging that social norms and expectations for medicine have always been in transition, such as an increased focus on dealing with illness experiences, the importance of holistic, healing interactions with clinicians and providers, and wellness and health promotion as goals (Ritvo et al., 1999; Truant and McKenzie, 1999). A focus on organ function, biological markers, and disease-related variables is restrictive and is no longer an adequate reflection of the social values of patients or the public's expectations for effective health care (Glik, 2000; Jonas, 1998; Mike, 1999; Thorne at al., 2002). Importantly, recent studies suggest that some conventional physicians no longer conceive of their practices as limited by their biomedical training and that some practitioners are discussing, referring to or practicing some of the more prominent forms of CAM and believe them to be useful or efficacious (Astin, 1998).

Yet, care must be taken not to assume compatibility where none exists. Medical pluralism should be distinguished from the cooptation of CAM therapies by conventional medical practices (Kaptchuk and Eisenberg, 2001). Although some conventional medical practices may seek and achieve a genuine integration with various CAM therapies, the hazard of integration is that certain CAM therapies may be delivered within the context of a conventional medical practice in ways that dissociate CAM modalities from the epistemological framework that guides the tailoring of the CAM practice. If this occurs, the healing process is likely to be less effective or even ineffective, undermining both the CAM therapy and the conventional biomedical practice. This is especially the case when the impact or change intended by the CAM therapy relies on a notion of efficacy that is not readily measurable by current scientific means.

A commitment to medical pluralism also has major implications for how research is conducted. Howard Brody puts the problem succinctly: "Therapies that might be highly effective within the proper cultural and belief context might prove to be totally ineffective within the foreign environment required for and created by the conduct of an RCT [randomized controlled trial]" (Brody, 2002). Thus, medical pluralism requires a commitment to finding innovative ways to assess efficacy, in accord with its multiple meanings and the diverse contexts in which it may occur.

In sum, the practice of medical pluralism will mean moving beyond any medicocentric claims for the ultimate ability of biomedicine to incorporate all CAM therapies that are of use while discarding the rest. This will require suspending any categorical disbelief in CAM therapies, at least long enough to consider the evidence for safety and efficacy dispassionately (and sometimes innovatively) and in their appropriate contexts rather than only within the framework of conventional medicine practice or the usual scientific norms. Thus, the committee suggests that the proper attitude is one of skepticism about any claim that conventional biomedical research and practice exhaustively account for the human experiences of health and healing, combined with diligent efforts to discern the significance, safety, and efficacy of CAM therapies.

5. The first four ethical commitments (to personal and public beneficence, to protection, to patient autonomy and consumer choice, and to medical pluralism in the service of these aims) provide the general framework for this chapter and inform the committee's selection of areas that require more extensive exploration. In explicitly stating these commitments, the committee also implies a fifth commitment, namely, *public accountability*, both for this report and its findings and for the health care system in the United States. Were medical research and health care a private matter paid for by private funds and with few social consequences, such public accountability would not be required. Yet, health care, as well as the medical research that supports it, is a public trust that is largely funded with common resources and that has broad societal consequences. Accountability to the public for prudent and fair assessment and use of medical and health care resources is a necessary component of this report.

The committee recognizes the complexity of a commitment to public accountability for CAM therapies. For example, many consumers access CAM therapies outside the context of primary or other medical care; pay for such therapies out of pocket; do not consult with their physicians regarding such care; and use CAM therapies for relaxation, wellness, spiritual awareness, or reasons other than biomedical disease management (Eisenberg et al., 1993, 1998). Similarly, many CAM therapies are offered as part of a healing process that involves meaning and is attentive to the illness experience and perceptions of risk and vulnerability. Many CAM providers regard their therapeutic regimens to be other than and outside systems of conventional medical care, reimbursement, or even licensure, and are concerned with healing as distinct from curing (Young, 1982; Eisenberg et al., 2002). The question of whether licensure, reimbursement, and inclusion within hospital-based, integrative models of care would be a socially desired good or an undesirable compromise (or even a dilution of healing traditions) becomes especially significant when one considers that prayer, meditation, and other forms of spiritual healing exist within the rubric of CAM therapies. For many CAM providers offering services in these domains (and their patients), the significance of a given therapeutic intervention may be less about efficacy on the physiological level and more about emotional health, coping, psychological growth, transformation, and self-actualization (Maslow, 1968). Likewise, therapeutic efficacy may involve such arguably vague but no less powerful spiritual themes as reconciliation with the divine or other formulations of "at-one-ment" and wholeness, or simply, perhaps, a renewed or more expanded sense of self (Astin and Astin, 2002). Stated in these terms, providers offering (and clients availing themselves of) some of these therapies may focus less on the kind of physiological results validated by evidence in medicine and public health and more on intangible, yet nonetheless compelling, personal benefits. Such services may have less kinship with technologically oriented, biomedical interventions and greater kinship with therapies at the borderland of psychological and spiritual care that are offered in professions such as pastoral counseling and hospice.

Stated slightly differently, by virtue of their overtly psychological or spiritual aspirations, some of these therapies may have less to do with outer results and may have more to do with a kind of "inner revolution." For example, Robert Thurman links inner spiritual evolution and outer social change through Tibetan Buddhist psychological and religious teachings (Thurman, 1998). In the Western traditions, philosophers and religious thinkers as diverse as Plato and Mary Baker Eddy have ascribed to linkages between health and various ritual practices, beliefs, or ways of thinking. Thus, although physicians or public health professionals may speak in terms of morbidity, mortality, and risk factors, other kinds of clinicians and therapists may think in terms of healing the shadow self and increasing the capacity for intimacy and mature love (Fromm-Reichmann, 1960) or the growth of (and care for) the soul (Ingerman, 1991). Some physicians would even link these two domains (Ornish, 1998). In other words, public accountability, like medical pluralism, must include some consideration of the vast array of perspectives that constitute the national (and even international) heritage of healing traditions.

In this light, some CAM providers would prefer that their healing traditions remain outside conventional systems of care and reimbursement and beyond the reach of efforts at integration (Cohen, 1998; Eisenberg et al., 1998). The complexity and persistence of such issues are evident not only in the domain of licensure and credentialing but also in the domain of herbal products. Questions have arisen, for example, who *can* own the knowledge of indigenous herbal traditions; who *should* own such knowledge; and under what conditions (or even whether at all) may such knowledge be transferred, developed, commercialized, or maintained as private (or in some traditions, sacred, and thereby beyond public dissemination)?

Such questions also touch on the nature of scientific evidence and whether methodologies appropriate to these issues of accountability can be designed.

An additional complicating factor in public accountability is that companies that have successfully marketed a CAM product may have not only philosophical reservations but also little or no financial incentive to have their product tested in independent settings. Perhaps only those companies that strongly believe in their products and that are willing to risk the revealing of evidence contrary to their convictions about their products (and those of loyal practitioners and customers) would willingly participate in research on their products. An additional financial disincentive is the difficulty in securing a patent on many of these products. Yet, insofar as these products are part of health care practices and are labeled or used as such by the American public, the manner is which they are regulated should account for all five of the ethical commitments outlined here, including accountability.

Accountability thus includes a sensitivity to the complex needs and desires of multiple constituents within the public sector (e.g., licensed clinicians and other healers, patients, professional organizations, regulatory boards, and other government authorities) and at the same time a recognition of the heterogeneity of communities and interests within each set of constituents (e.g., multiple regulatory boards with overlapping or intersecting authorities; multiple professional groups with competing theories, definitions of practice, lineages of tradition, and legislative goals; multiple patient and consumer protection groups, each balancing the paternalism-autonomy dilemma in different ways; and multiple stakeholders within the federal government and state governments). Accountability also includes a sensitivity to the blurring of boundaries that increasingly occurs not only between the legally authorized scope of practice for different professions (for example, the overlap between professions such as chiropractic, physical therapy, and massage therapy) (Cohen, 1998) but also between emerging (or frontier) practices in medicine, the mental health professions, CAM professions that use bioenergetic or biofield approaches to therapy (NIH, 1995; Jonas and Chez, 2003), and various forms of spiritual care (Cohen, 2003). For example, hypnosis and guided imagery are related therapies that may cross the chasm between the physical and the metaphysical realms, as both can be used for different purposes by surgeons, dentists, and massage therapists, as well as in clinics for smoking cessation and weight loss and in hospice. Moreover, therapeutic goals can range from pain reduction and accelerated healing to the kind of growth envisioned in fields such as transpersonal psychology (Rosen, 1982). Sensitivity to all the complexities described above will be evident in the committee's approach, the ethical commitments highlighted, and the recommendations.

VALUE JUDGMENTS IN DEFINING CAM

Value judgments are implicit in the term CAM itself. Just deciding what should be categorized as a CAM therapy—as distinct from a religious ritual or a cultural practice—from among the dozens of alternative practices is a decision with important value implications. The reasons for defining modalities as "CAM therapies" are not only scientific but also political, social, and conceptual (Jonas, 2002). These include a lack of a generally accepted explanatory model; the fact that the origin of the practice (e.g., acupuncture) is outside of the dominant system; the amount of data or the type of data is considered insufficient or otherwise inadequate (e.g., herbalism and megavitamin therapy); the use of the practice is marginalized in that it is not widely available within conventional hospitals (e.g., chiropractic); the teaching of the practice is marginalized in that it is not generally taught within medical, nursing, or graduate schools of the dominant institutions (e.g., nutritional therapy); the amount of research funding, infrastructure, and capacity for investigating the practice is low (e.g., massage); reimbursement for the practice is not provided by insurance companies and third-party payers; the practice is not readily used for feasibility, acceptability, or other reasons (e.g., clinical ecology and complex lifestyle programs); the practice is not regulated or licensed in most states (e.g., naturopathy); and an aspect of the therapy is marginalized, even though it is studied under other names or subdivisions (e.g., antineoplastons and shark cartilage). In brief, when something is labeled "CAM": and when "CAM therapies" are sorted and differentiated, it is important to recognize the diverse social and political value judgments at work. These value judgments are sometimes embedded in the scientific, medical, and educational rationales for health taxonomies. Attending to these implicit value components will reduce the likelihood of miscategorization and misunderstanding.

The following sections address three sets of ethical issues in CAM research and practice: ethical issues in CAM research; ethical issues in the integration of CAM therapies into conventional practice; and related legal and regulatory issues. Some of the conclusions from this chapter are included in the recommendations of other chapters of the report. An additional aim of this chapter is to raise questions and flag areas that practitioners, researchers, and policy makers believe will need to be considered in greater depth.

ETHICAL ISSUES IN CAM RESEARCH

Over the past 60 years the major sources for guidance on the ethics of research with human subjects in the United States have been the Nuremberg Code (1946), the Declaration of Helsinki (1964, revised in 1996), the International Ethical Guidelines for Biomedical Research Involving Human Subjects (1982, revised in 1993), the Belmont Report of the National Commission for the Protection of Human Subjects in Biomedical and Behavioral Research (1979), and the federal Common Rule, (U.S. Department of Health and Human Services, 45 CFR 46, 1991). Emanuel and colleagues (2000) have proposed a consolidation and synthesis of the diverse principles and norms in these various codes and statements into seven requirements which, if satisfied, "make clinical research ethical." Their synthesis provides a useful beginning point for considering the ethical challenges raised by CAM research.

Social or Scientific Value

The value of a research project is the extent to which it holds the promise of improving health or increasing knowledge important to health, when it is judged on either social or scientific grounds. Social or scientific value must be considered because resources available for research are scarce and should be expended wisely. It is also ethically imperative that subjects enrolled in clinical trials not be placed at risk except in the search for socially or scientifically important results. The placement of subjects at risk for an insignificant outcome is exploitation. Here the challenge for CAM research will be to select for investigation those therapies that have the greatest social or scientific significance. Yet, CAM therapies do not constitute a consistent or unified set of practices but constitute a wide-ranging set of highly variable practices, valued in different ways by the constituencies that deliver and receive them. This is a difference in degree, but not in kind, from the decisions that policy makers and researchers already face, for example, when they are faced with decisions about whether to fund more research on hypertension, cancer, or depression. Such decisions, however, may be more complex when CAM therapies are considered, precisely because there may be no common standard for adjudicating the relative value of various CAM therapies, except perhaps by recourse to conventional biomedical definitions and rankings of health and disease. Yet exclusive recourse to conventional definitions and rankings would challenge the commitment to pluralism. Thus, even in the selection of which CAM remedies to investigate, there is the need for negotiation about the relative social and scientific values of therapies. There is also a risk, common to many areas of medical research, that the commercial interest of providers and manufacturers will dominate over public interests and health needs (Hilts, 2003). Ensuring that social and scientific values prevail over commercial ones will be an ongoing ethical task.

Scientific Validity

Validity results when scientific principles and methods are used to produce reliable outcomes. Ethically, the same considerations that endorse social or scientific value also underwrite scientific validity. Research that is underpowered, that does not have a testable hypothesis, or that cannot otherwise achieve its purpose is a waste of resources and constitutes the exploitation of human subjects, who are placed at risk for no beneficial purpose. For CAM research, it is important to ask about the range of scientific validity that is appropriate and what should count as a validated therapy. Because it entails social values, this is as much an ethical as an epistemological question. For example, should a "validated therapy" mean one that can be adequately explained in terms of the conventional biomedical model or, more simply, one that can be shown to provide benefit, even in the absence of a scientific explanation of its mechanism of action? Ethically, this presents a value-based choice between a more conventional scientific understanding of a validated CAM therapy and a more pragmatic stance that may not be consistent with current research standards for conventional medicine. In a parallel but slightly different context, regulations such as disciplinary provisions in medical licensing statues that divide the world of CAM therapies into such categories as "validated," "invalidated," and "nonvalidated" and do so partly in terms of theoretical "plausibility" should also be examined for both epistemological and ethical assumptions.

Fair Subject Selection

The ethical principle at play in fair subject selection is justice. Putting justice to work in clinical research means selecting subjects so that there is an equitable distribution of benefits and burdens. This means attending to the relative vulnerability of subjects for certain kinds of high-risk research, making sure that there is equity in subject selection along the lines of racial-ethnic socioeconomic status, gender, and other factors. More generally, fair subject selection means that those who bear the risks of research should be among those who reap the benefits and that those populations who enjoy the fruits of research should also share in the risks. There is no simple formula for how to achieve fair subject selection, but there are federal requirements both for protecting certain categories of vulnerable populations (e.g., pregnant women, children, and prisoners) and for including women and children unless they are inappropriate to the study. If CAM therapies generally were used predominantly by indigent populations or by certain ethnic or racial minorities, justice would require, other things being equal, that the subject populations be drawn from these groups and that these groups be among the first to receive whatever benefits were available from any newly validated therapies. The United States has yet to enact policies that ensure justice in the distribution of the fruits of research, even for conventional medical research. The stipulation of such goals for CAM would be a good precedent, although awaiting the adoption of such standards of justice will require major policy changes and the absence of such standards should not delay research on CAM.

Favorable Risk-Benefit Ratios

The ethical norm of risk-benefit contains several principles, some of which were discussed above. These include the obligation to minimize risks to subjects during the trial (nonmaleficence), to enhance potential benefits (beneficence), and to ensure that the benefits to subjects or society, or both, are worth the risks incurred (proportionality and nonexploitation). For many CAM practices the absence of standardization among practitioners, combined with imprecise measures of outcomes, could make the risk-benefit ratio more difficult to assess when subjects are enrolled in a trial and thereby make the informed-consent process more vague and fragile. For example, many CAM therapies emphasize a concept of wellness that is more holistic and inclusive than typical outcomes research. Whether and how to include this more imprecise aspect of health into a clinical trial is a question of both epistemology and ethics, that is, both the research methodology and the ends that are valued and sought through research.

Informed Consent

Considered by many as the heart of research ethics, informed consent expresses the obligation of researchers to inform potential subjects of the purpose of research, its risks and benefits, along with the alternatives, in a manner that ensures that the participants understand these elements of research and can act freely to enroll or decline. Informed consent is one of the chief ways of promoting subject autonomy, or self-determination, which is the right of free choice based on one's own values. Some of those designated as vulnerable in the federal Common Code are categorized as such precisely because of their diminished capacity to give consent. More generally, it is now well recognized that subjects who are ill and who participate in research in a clinical setting, often with their regular doctors acting as researchers, are likewise in a vulnerable position with regard to informed consent (Appelbaum et al., 1987; U.S. Advisory Committee on Human Radiation Experiments, 1996). Here the issue is not subjects' mental capacities, but their expectations, with the subjects often attributing more therapeutic potential to a research project than the evidence or the trial design warrants. This has been termed the "therapeutic misconception," and it is a known hazard for both subjects and investigators, and perhaps also for others in the research process, such as sponsors and institutional review boards (IRBs) (Dresser, 2002; Henderson and King, 2003; Miller, 2000). It may be an especially vexing issue for trials involving CAM therapies, especially those CAM therapies that rely on the expectancy of patients or on close practitioner-patient relationships for a substantial part of their efficacy.

In other words, working to correct the therapeutic misconception in clinical trials of CAM therapies may undermine precisely those elements of belief and expectancy on which some CAM therapies rely. Therefore, care should be taken to design protocols that can take account of this component of expectancy (without vitiating it). In this regard CAM therapies differ only in degree, and not in kind, from research with conventional remedies. Investigators and sponsors should be vigilant about expectancy factors in themselves, as well as in subjects and in the informed consent process as CAM therapies are tested.

Independent Review

Independent review means a review of the research design, subject population, risk-benefit ratio, and so forth, by persons with expertise in these facets of research and not affiliated with the trial in question. The aim here is to minimize conflicts of interests, ensure objectivity, and enhance public accountability. Independent review of CAM trials may pose challenges in terms of finding reviewers who are knowledgeable about the modalities under investigation and about research procedures and yet who are sufficiently disinterested about the outcomes.

Respect for Potential and Enrolled Subjects

This last, catchall category of respect incorporates several requirements: (1) permitting subject withdrawal from the research; (2) protecting subject privacy through confidentiality; (3) informing subjects of changes in risks and benefits during the trial; (4) making the research results available to the subjects of that research; and (5) generally, maintaining the welfare of the subjects throughout the trial. Here CAM therapies pose a potential issue of expertise in research oversight. Typically, IRBs consist of individuals with knowledge and expertise in conventional medicine modalities and research. Thus, it will be necessary to identify and recruit reviewers who have knowledge of CAM therapies and who are well versed in both the standard protocols and any innovative features involved in CAM protocols.

Beyond these more particular areas for ethical inquiry, it is important to acknowledge the powerful role of social perceptions and values in shaping biomedical research policy. These perceptions and values will likely be at play in CAM research as well and may perhaps be at play in more pronounced ways. In the 1970s, when ethical guidelines and federal regulations governing clinical research were first codified, research was generally conceived of as a risky undertaking from which subjects needed protection. The late 1980s and early 1990s marked a major shift in public and scientific attitudes toward research "from protection to access" (Churchill et al., 1998; Mastroianni and Kahn, 2001). AIDS activism played a major role in this transition; eagerness to participate in clinical trials is now a common occurrence, even for Phase I research, in which the chances for benefit are remote or nonexistent (Daugherty et al., 1995, 2000). Some practitioners, patients, and policy makers regard all clinical research to be presumptively beneficial, so that being denied access to a trial is considered discrimination (King, 1995). In this climate, there is a need to consider carefully a balance that will "reconcile public safety with public demand" (Thorne et al., 2002). When public demand is fueled by commercial and entrepreneurial interests, as has been the case in gene therapy research, the task of achieving balance can be difficult (Churchill et al., 1998; Orkin and Motulsky, 1995; Ross et al., 1996). This is an ongoing challenge for all medical research, but it is a particularly important one for CAM research, especially research on those CAM modalities in which public assumptions about efficacy are prevalent and for which commercial forces are strong.

In summary CAM therapies should be rigorously evaluated for reasons of both public safety and health promotion. The ethical principles that guide conventional biomedical research should also be applied to CAM research (Miller et al., 2004). Yet, careful attention will be required to discern the applicability of these principles; and some of the key terms, such as "informed consent," "equipoise," and "risk-benefit" will sometimes have interpretations in CAM research different from those in research conducted by conventional medical protocols.

ETHICAL ISSUES IN THE INTEGRATION OF CAM THERAPIES INTO CONVENTIONAL MEDICAL PRACTICE

Although the major sources for modern research ethics have all been created within the past 60 years, some of the chief ethical precepts for conventional clinical practice enjoy a 2,500-year history. All Western ethical traditions for medical practice trace their origins to the Hippocratic Oath (sixth century B.C.E.), and many graduates of U.S. medical schools still mark their commencement with a recitation of some version of this oath. More recent ethical guidelines for medical practice can be found in Maimonides' Daily Prayer for a Physician (1793), the American Medical Associations' first Code of Ethics (1847) and its more recent Principles

(2001), and the Declaration of Geneva (1948). In addition, most of the recognized specialty organizations of U.S. conventional medicine have adopted their own codes, principles, or guidelines to address ethical issues germane to their work.

It is clear from even a cursory look that the official, written codes of CAM practitioners indicate a parallel set of commitments and many similar principles and virtues. For example, the *Code of Ethics* of the American Chiropractic Association includes duties of confidentiality, privacy, and loyalty; obligations not to neglect or abandon the patient; duties of honesty and competency; and the use of modalities that are in the patient's best interest and not in conflict with applicable statutory or administrative rules (ACA, 1996). Duties of confidentiality, nonabandonment, and competency are also reflected in ethical codes and manuals for physicians (American College of Physicians, 1998).

Similarly, the *Model Code of Ethics* of the Acupuncture and Oriental Medicine Commission requires, among other things, that practitioners be competent, maintain patient confidences and records, not abandon patients, provide a clear treatment plan, charge fees that are not excessive, inform the patient regarding contraindications, maintain appropriate therapeutic boundaries, and refrain from false or misleading advertising (NAFTA Acupuncture and Oriental Medicine Commission, 1997). Likewise, the *Naturopathic Code of Ethics* of the American Association of Naturopathic Physicians includes nonmaleficence among its guiding principles to "provide the most effective health care available with the least risk to his/her patients at all times" and requires that naturopathic physicians maintain competence and honesty (AANP, 1990).

These common aims regarding patient care and practitioner duties should provide some initial common ground for the negotiations about when and how practicioners can collaborate or integrate forms of care while respecting the pluralism necessary to sustain what is valuable and distinctive within each system of care.

Nevertheless, the effort to integrate CAM therapies into conventional medicine practice can present the physician with a variety of ethical challenges. Given the prevalence of CAM use by the general public it is clear that many patients seen in conventional medical clinics are also seeing CAM providers or using CAM therapies. This presents the conventional medicine practitioner not only with opportunities of defining physician-patient relationships in new ways and with expanded understandings of "health" and "care" but also with some new responsibilities and some potential hazards regarding patient safety and adherence to physician recommendations. For example, it is now important that conventional medicine practitioners ask about a patient's use of CAM when the patient's history is taken. Such history taking must be done in a safe environment in which the patient can freely discuss the CAM therapies that he or she has received or is receiving without fear of punitive judgment or the withdrawal of conventional medical care. A moral correlate to this elicitation is the physician's obligation to be well informed about the CAM modalities most frequently used by patients, an obligation of candor about the physician's level of knowledge of the CAM modalities in question, and, following from that, an obligation to make patients aware of whatever safety and efficacy information is available (Eisenberg, 1997; Sugarman and Burk, 1998). Ernst and Cohen (2001) discuss this as the duty "to tell patients about the degree of uncertainty associated with the efficacy and safety of the treatment, as well as the availability and risk-benefit ratio of other treatment options." However, this is further complicated by the conventional medicine practitioners' limited exposure to CAM modalities, lack of knowledge about CAM, minimal or nonexistent educational tools, and limited access to resources, as well as the current practice demands on conventional medicine practitioners. In these interactions, ethics will require a balancing of principles and commitments. Any decision to forgo conventional medical treatment should be accompanied by careful monitoring of the patient by the conventional practitioner (Cohen and Eisenberg, 2002; Ernst and Cohen, 2001).

Adams and colleagues (2002) presented a helpful delineation of options for the physician in recommending, tolerating, or in some cases, actively proscribing CAM therapies to patients on the basis of an individualized risk-benefit assessment. The ethical analysis suggested for the clinical consideration of the use of a CAM therapy involves weighing the severity and the acuteness of illness; the curability of the illness by conventional forms of medical treatment; the degree of invasiveness, associated toxicities, and side effects of the conventional medical treatment; the availability and quality of evidence of the utility and safety of the CAM treatment; the level of understanding of the risks and the benefits of the CAM treatment, combined with the patient's knowledge and voluntary acceptance of those risks; and the patient's persistence of intention to use the CAM therapies. Evaluation of all these factors can be very helpful in analyzing particular cases and inevitably involves a scaling and balancing of the ethical norms discussed above. The implications for physician action based on their "risk framework" can be summarized as follows:

> If evidence [concerning the CAM therapy] supports both safety and efficacy, the physician should recommend the therapy but continue to monitor the patient conventionally. If evidence supports safety but is inconclusive about efficacy, the treatment should be cautiously tolerated and monitored for effectiveness. If evidence supports efficacy but is inconclusive about safety, the therapy could still be tolerated and monitored for safety. Finally, therapies for which evidence indicates either serious risk or ineffi-

cacy obviously should be avoided and patients actively discouraged from pursuing such a course of treatment. (Adams et al., 2002)

These recommendations are sound, but they raise further questions about how they can be carried out. Many CAM therapies have not been systematically researched, and the information available may be limited and not within the practicing physician's fund of knowledge. Medical education for students and residents as well as for physicians in private practice will need to be addressed and revised so that physicians can fulfill these new obligations for their patient populations. Realistically, this will take significant effort, time, and resources, as well as a commitment to ensure that CAM modalities can be effectively discussed with and framed appropriately for patients, as Adams and colleagues have outlined.

Some argue that there is enough agreement in basic aims between conventional medicine and CAM to permit CAM practices to be embraced, so long as the therapies that they offer are safe and effective. For example, Sugarman and Burk (1998) compared the health-related goals of a standard list of conventional medicine and CAM practices and found commonality in terms of prevention, relief of pain and suffering, care for those who cannot be cured, and general promotion and maintenance of health (Bratman, 1997; Callahan, 1996; Sugarman and Burk, 1998). Yet beyond these formal commonalities are deeper questions about the methods and means by which these health-related goals are reached. Moreover, the expanding use of CAM practitioners and therapies implies a sense of the limits of conventional medicine and conventional medical practice in accomplishing its desired health goals, even if the conventional therapies are not perceived as inadequate by the public. Callahan (1996) poses the question this way: "What is lacking in conventional medicine that they [patients] seek?" Put more pointedly, "Why do so many people in the U.S. pay out-of-pocket to see CAM practitioners and use CAM remedies?" At least a partial answer has been identified by Astin, who concluded that CAM providers seem to have norms and styles of interaction with patients that are more congruent with patients "values, beliefs, and philosophical orientations toward health and life." The reasons for the widespread and growing use of CAM therapies are many, but for Astin, one reason, arguably, is the public's desire for a kind of health service and a kind of patient-provider interaction that is sometimes not available through the services offered by conventional medicine. Further research comparing conventional medicine and CAM practitioners on biopsychosocial dimensions in the delivery of health services would be useful both for medical research and medical practice.

Although it seems likely that conventional medicine can be enhanced through the study of CAM practices, it is neither possible nor desirable for conventional medicine to adopt all salutary features of high-quality CAM care. On some occasions, and for some individuals, CAM practices are indeed distinctive and truly complementary to conventional medicine, especially when the CAM practitioner and patient share a cultural heritage or a spiritual tradition. In these cases, most physicians will possess neither the skills nor the inclination to learn and incorporate CAM practices, and indeed, integration into a single practice norm should not be the aim. However, it is also possible, and perhaps even desirable, for patients-consumers that some proven CAM practices be incorporated into conventional medicine, for example, acupuncture for chemotherapy-induced nausea. To do so would be in keeping with commitments to beneficence, nonmaleficence, and respect for patient autonomy, as well as the best caring traditions of all health professionals. Yet, as noted earlier, integration also runs the risk of co-optation. It is also possible that referral to an acupuncture practitioner be made to offer these patients this service without integrating acupuncture into the conventional medical practice. Integration is not always desirable, and even when it is desirable, may not be feasible. The meaning and aim of "integration" requires a careful definition, clarity around the value assumptions that it entails, and negotiation about the epistemic and political assumptions that it carries, in addition to its more immediate patient care goals.

RELATED LEGAL AND REGULATORY ISSUES

Ethical concerns in clinical care, whether they involve conventional or CAM therapies, frequently overlap with legal considerations. For example, the obligation to provide adequate informed consent has both ethical and legal dimensions and, whether involving biomedical or CAM therapies, requires disclosure of all information material to a treatment decision (Ernst and Cohen, 2001). This includes the probability that the patient will benefit from the procedure, the probability that the patient will encounter risks associated with this procedure, and the alternative options that are feasible and available as well as their risks and benefits (Ernst and Cohen, 2001). Thus, if a reasonable physician (or a reasonable patient, depending on the state) finds that a program that incorporates yoga, meditation, and lifestyle changes for the prevention and treatment of cardiac disease is material to a treatment decision (or that *Gingko biloba* improves dementia because of circulation problems or possibly Alzheimer's disease [Kleinjen and Knipschild, 1992; LeBars et al., 1997]), then the clinician is ethically and legally required to discuss the risks and benefits of the program (or dietary supplement) (Cohen, 2000; Ernst and Cohen, 2001). This requirement is in keeping with the contemporary shift toward shared decision making between patient and clinician, in which patient preferences are actively considered and valued. This is resonant with a baseline commitment to patient autonomy. Attending to patient preferences is not only morally laudatory, because it is part of honoring patient self-determination, but also may increase adherence and, by that means, efficacy as well.

Questions will inevitably arise about just how much evidence about a CAM therapy is needed before it becomes a part of the treatment options routinely mentioned or offered to patients. It can be argued that it is unethical to offer any CAM therapy until evidence from an RCT is complete. The stronger argument is that judgments about how much evidence is enough must be referenced to a diversity of factors, including the efficacies of conventional medical therapies; the hazards of the CAM modalities in question, if any; the extent to which these CAM modalities are preferred by patients; and the overall quality of whatever evidence exists. It should not be forgotten that RCTs of many conventional medical therapies that are routinely recommended and widely used have not been conducted. Posing the RCT as the sole test and necessary barrier for acceptance of a CAM therapy is questionable and may not be applicable with respect to certain CAM modalities. Requiring RCTs may undermine the commitment to medical pluralism.

As noted above, Adams and colleagues (2002) offer a helpful framework for addressing the therapeutic relationship in the absence of significant evidence, when there is no standard efficacious treatment or when conventional therapy has failed, and when the patient's intention to use a CAM therapy is strong and persistent. When the implications of this framework are spelled out and the patient makes an informed, autonomous choice in favor a CAM therapy, it may, indeed, be unethical for the physician to withhold either treatment or an appropriate referral (Adams et al., 2002; Cohen, 2003). The rationale is that, as a general rule, "the personal beliefs and choices of other persons should be respected if they pose no threat to other parties" (Adams et al., 2002). If a patient with a precancerous condition, for example, seeks to pursue such therapies as meditation, colonics, yoga, and reiki rather than surgery for a limited time while continuing monitoring by a physician, it is ethically compelling for the physician to honor the patient's core values and internal sense of integrity while compassionately discussing the physician's perspective (Adams et al., 2002). The physician who cannot in good conscience support this choice can document informed refusal of care and needs to consider the caring commitment that is part of the ongoing relationship with the patient (Adams et al., 2002). Such a physician may feel that it is medically incorrect, given his or her training and experience, to elect to support the patient's preference for CAM; and even though the physician is compassionate, he or she may be unable to administer or support care effectively. The ethical obligation of nonabandonment requires that if the physician opts to withdraw from care, referral to a more like-minded physician who can continue to monitor the patient is warranted (Adams et al., 2002).

Although physicians should be clear about the ethical duty of nonabandonment, they should also "take the initiative to proactively steer the patient away from treatments that are known to be dangerous or have been associated with clinically significant adverse interactions with other supplements or medications" (Adams et al., 2002). Moreover, when there is no evidence either for or against a given CAM therapy, physicians "can choose to tolerate and monitor or actively discourage use of CAM treatments" (Adams et al., 2002; Cohen and Eisenberg, 2002). In so doing, physicians should consider such factors as the severity and acuteness of the illness; the manageability or curability of the illness by conventional forms of treatment; the degree of invasiveness, associated toxicities, and side effects of the conventional treatment; the availability and quality of evidence of the utility and safety of the desired CAM treatment; the level of understanding of the risks and benefits of the CAM treatment combined with the patient's knowledge and voluntary acceptance of those risks; and the patient's persistence of intention to use CAM therapies (Adams et al., 2002). By following this procedure, clinicians can formulate a plan that is "clinically sound, ethically appropriate, and targeted to the unique circumstances of individual patients" even in the absence of scientific evidence (Adams et al., 2002). The ensuing discussions between physicians and patients not only are the "heart of informed consent," but also are "often the beginning rather than the ending" of the conversation (Adams et al., 2002). The best approach should take into consideration the unique circumstances of the individual patient. While some tension between medical pluralism and an evidence-based approach is likely inevitable and probably productive, the committee suggests that some of this tension can be resolved by CAM research and that the concept of evidence-based medicine will need to be modified to accommodate the multiple approaches inherent within a pluralistic understanding of health care.

Finally, when a clinician decides whether to offer, recommend, discourage, or accept a patient's use of CAM therapies or refer patients to CAM providers, ethical obligations and legal duties (or at least liability considerations) may diverge (Cohen, 2003). For instance, it may be legal, but perhaps not ethical, for a physician with minimum training in acupuncture to provide the patient such treatment (Cohen, 2003). Conversely, it may be ethically compelling, but legally risky, to have an unbiased discussion with a terminally ill patient who is suffering from an incurable brain tumor yet who is ineligible for available clinical trials and who is interested in trying a treatment not accepted as safe and effective by the Food and Drug Administration (Cohen, 2003; U.S. House of Representatives, 1996; *United States v. Rutherford*, 1979). In this situation the physician may face a conflict of values or at least a worldview divergent from that of the patient, who may not share with the physician an understanding of the role and the value of scientific evidence (or the lack thereof) with the same intensity. Any collision of values requires sensitivity to the patient's expression of interests that goes well beyond the legalistic requirements of informed consent, as well as attention to the malleable but important fabric of the therapeutic encounter. In this respect, the ethical commitment to medical pluralism should be considered as the physician wrestles with conversations involving patient decision making.

Similarly, a physician may ethically support a patient's stated desire to try yoga, colonics, or reiki for a limited period rather than surgery, yet the clinician might be concerned about potential liability if he or she accepts the patient's choice (Adams et al., 2002). Alternatively, the clinician may be sensitive to the potential for unwarranted professional discipline, based on the use of therapies not generally accepted within the profession (Cohen, 1998). Likewise, a hospital administrator may wish to limit potential liability exposure by introducing only those CAM therapies that have been demonstrated to be safe and effective to the satisfaction of a hospital committee, the Food and Drug Administration, or a medical specialty group; yet ethically, denying patients access to a larger range of therapies could conceivably contravene interests in beneficence (e.g., by depriving patients of potential therapeutic benefit), justice (e.g., by ensuring access to therapies), and autonomy (e.g., respecting the patient's interest in therapies and choice of treatment). As well, once a therapy becomes generally medically accepted, failure to provide adequate informed consent can result in potential malpractice liability (Ernst and Cohen, 2001; *Moore v. Baker*, 1993).

On a broader level, legal and ethical issues often arise, and sometimes conflict, with CAM therapies because the decision facing a clinician (or institution) may engender a conflict between medical paternalism (the desire to protect patients from foolish or ill-informed, although voluntary, decisions) and patient autonomy (Cohen 1998, 2003). As suggested, the conflict between paternalism and autonomy can be accentuated by the patient's selection of therapies that may, at the moment of choice, lack general medical acceptance or a sufficiently recognized evidentiary base (Cohen, 2003a). Whether strong paternalism—which would violate a patient's informed, voluntary, and autonomous choice—is justified depends on a number of factors, including the possibility that the projected benefits of the paternalistic action will outweigh its risks to the patient and the possibility that the least autonomy-restrictive alternative that will secure the benefits and reduce the risks is selected (Beauchamp and Childress, 1994; Cohen, 1995, 1998). Yet, the exercise of strong paternalism should be a rare event (even if it is not so rare in practice), and patient autonomy (for competent adults) is the presumptive norm for all medical care. This is because achieving genuine patient autonomy always involves information giving, discussion with the patient, and other enabling actions. Precisely because it involves dialogue on perspectives other than those of the provider, including interpreting the facts and probing the meaning of choices, autonomy for patients normally implies the best standard for medical decision making. The challenge for practitioners in achieving and honoring such autonomy may well be greater when patients are considering CAM therapies than when they are considering conventional medical therapies. Practitioners not only may have less information about CAM modalities, but they also may be uncomfortable in the discussion of CAM therapies, since information on CAM is often couched in more analogical and metaphorical language than the mechanistic cause-and-effect imagery typical of the remedies offered by conventional medicine.

Regulatory structures increasingly acknowledge the need for weighing and balancing of differing standards. For example, *Model Guidelines for the Use of Complementary and Alternative Therapies in Medical Practice*, promulgated by the Federation of State Medical Boards (FSMB, 2002), explicitly allow for "a wide latitude in physicians' exercise of their professional judgment," recognize that "patients have a right to seek any kind of care for their health problems," and aim to create rules that are "clinically responsible and ethically appropriate." Although the model guidelines as a whole may or may not balance or even explicitly address the five ethical commitments enumerated earlier, the quoted language at least establishes a greater balance between physician and patient preferences than has historically been supposed. Similarly states are considering whether revisions to their own medical disciplinary provisions require amendment to more appropriately balance one or more of the ethical commitments outlined earlier in this chapter.

A number of legal rules also attempt to balance these competing interests and values and to protect patients by combating fraud and enhancing quality assurance while offering access to therapies and honoring medical pluralism in creating models of integrative care. Complex combinations of such rules may govern decisions by clinicians and health care institutions that seek to integrate CAM therapies into conventional medical settings (Cohen, 1998). In addition to informed consent, these rules include licensure and scope of practice, malpractice liability, professional discipline, food and drug law, health care fraud, and rules pertaining to third-party reimbursement (Cohen, 1998) and to spirituality in clinical settings (Cohen, 2003). These rules often work to elaborate and complement the five principal ethical commitments discussed at the beginning of this chapter: beneficence, nonmaleficence, protection and enablement of autonomy, medical pluralism, and public accountability. A brief discussion of these rules may be helpful, as they frequently dovetail with clinical decisions to recommend, tolerate or accept, or discourage patient use of CAM therapies and visits to CAM providers (Cohen and Eisenberg, 2002).

First, *licensure* is a matter of state law, since states have the power to license (or decline to license) any class of health care providers. This is because the Tenth Amendment to the U.S. Constitution provides that the powers not delegated to the federal government by the Constitution, nor prohibited by it to the states, are reserved to the states respectively, or to the people, and this reserved power includes regulation of health care licensure. In each state, the medical licensing statute (or medical practice act) prohibits the unlicensed practice of medicine, whereas other statutes license allied health professionals, such as nurses, physical therapists, and optometrists, and CAM providers such as chiropractors (Cohen, 1998; Eisenberg et al., 2002).

Licensure varies by state and profession, and ranges from mandatory licensure to title licensure and registration of the providers with a state agency (Cohen, 1998). Many CAM-related professional organizations are developing national standards for examination and licensure and legally authorized scopes of practice boundaries, ethics, and clinical practice (Eisenberg et al., 2002). Encouraging the continuing development and enhancement of such standards can help facilitate "collaboration and referral; offer more authoritative, consistent, and generalizable clinical and financial research; minimize access to unqualified CAM providers; and help . . . hospital credentialing and . . . risk management" (Eisenberg et al., 2002). Yet, "greater homogeneity may undermine the diversity of education, training, and skill, which historically have characterized many CAM professions," resulting in "excessive standardization, rigid scope of practice boundaries, excessive utilization standards . . . and fee schedules, increases in patient volume, decreases in individualization of services, a decrease in time spent per patient, and a perceived decrease in satisfaction by both patients and CAM practitioners" (Eisenberg et al., 2002). In any event, policies involving licensure, scope of practice and credentialing, and their relation to malpractice liability and risk management must be addressed creatively if health care institutions are to respond to patient interest in CAM therapies in ways that provide therapeutic benefit yet that satisfy liability concerns (Cohen and Ruggie, 2004).

Malpractice liability and *professional discipline* are intertwined, as a claim of negligence against a clinician could trigger civil liability through the former mechanism and the loss of licensure or some other sanction through the latter. In *Schneider v. Revici* the patient sued Dr. Revici for malpractice using a nutritional protocol to treat cancer. Dr. Revici offered a successful defense against the charge on the basis of the fact that the patient had signed an assumption of risk form (Cohen and Eisenberg, 2002). The caveat to this is that not all states accept assumption of risk as a defense, and its application can vary depending on the facts of the case. Likewise, a health care institution can be liable in malpractice cases for direct negligence (such as negligent credentialing or negligent failure to supervise a provider) or vicarious negligence (e.g., liability for the act of an employee or agent) (Cohen, 2000). Medical malpractice (negligence), whether it involves biomedical or CAM therapies, is generally defined as unskillful practice that fails to conform to a standard of care in the profession and that results in patient injury. CAM providers, like physicians and allied health care providers, can also be sued for negligence.

The application of liability (or discipline) becomes problematic if a conventional-medicine clinician's inclusion of CAM therapies is itself considered a deviation from prevailing and acceptable standards of care, as this could result in a conclusion of negligence, without necessarily finding evidence of wrongful conduct that caused patient injury (Cohen, 1999a,b, 2000). In *Charell v. Gonzales* the patient sued Dr. Gonzales for substituting a nutritional protocol for cancer care. The jury found Dr. Gonzales not only negligent but also reckless; however, the patient had implied consent to the protocol and, therefore, was deemed 49 percent responsible; liability was thus reduced accordingly (Cohen and Eisenberg, 2002). Once research establishes that a specific CAM therapy is within biomedical standards of care (e.g., the determination by a National Institutes of Health Consensus Panel that acupuncture is effective for the relief of nausea following chemotherapy [National Institutes of Health, 1997]), failure to recommend (or refer a patient for) such a therapy potentially could be considered malpractice (or could lead to professional discipline) if it results in patient injury (Cohen, 1998). In the case of *Moore v. Baker* (1993), a patient who received cardiac bypass surgery sued for malpractice, alleging inadequate informed consent because of the physician's failure to disclose the possibility of EDTA (ethylenediaminetetraacetic acid) chelation therapy as a less invasive alternative. The 11th Circuit Court held that if EDTA chelation therapy were generally accepted within the medical community, the patient might have an actionable claim.

As part of malpractice law, a nonphysician (whether he or she is an allied health care or CAM provider) has a legal (and ethical) duty to refer the patient to a medical doctor if the patient's condition exceeds the provider's training, skill, and competence or is not responding to the nonmedical treatment (Cohen, 1998). Similarly, the provider who makes a grossly exaggerated claim that induces reliance on a particular therapy potentially could be liable for fraud or misrepresentation (Cohen, 1998). Such legal rules frequently correspond with ethical provisions in the codes of some CAM professions and help protect patients against overzealous or overreaching practitioners (Cohen, 1998, 2000). It may be helpful for physicians to remember that CAM providers have a legal and ethical duty to refer a patient for conventional medical care when the patient's condition requires such referral.

Regarding referrals to CAM providers, the general legal rule is that physicians are not liable merely for referring the patient to another provider—whether that provider is a conventional medical or CAM practitioner—who turns out to be negligent. On the other hand, physician liability for "joint treatment" of the patient with a CAM provider, one notable exception to the general legal rule, may expand as integrative care results in greater coordination between biomedical and CAM providers (Cohen and Eisenberg, 2002) and the level of "claims consciousness" by patients of CAM providers increases (Studdert et al., 1998). Although such liability considerations continue to be unsettled, they should not necessarily preclude clinically sensible referrals, based on an awareness of what CAM providers can and cannot offer the patient, and a shared conversation regarding the objectives (and limits) of any one form of care (Cohen and Eisenberg, 2002). Such conversations, indeed, can help further a more pluralistic vision of health care, while offering the physician sufficient information to help navigate unwarranted liability concerns. Although clinicians and institutions can continue to be guided by considerations of safety and efficacy (Cohen and Eisenberg, 2002), as well as relevant ethical considerations (Adams et al., 2002), legal rules and institutions may continue to grow in their understanding of integrative health care practices as the field emerges.

Another emerging area, *food and drug law*, is complex and exists at the state as well as federal level. It also impacts the balance between paternalism and autonomy interest, as well the ethical commitment to medical pluralism. For example, Congress, in enacting the Dietary Supplement Health and Education Act (DSHEA), observed that the federal government "should not take any actions to impose unreasonable regulatory barriers limiting or slowing the flow of safe products and accurate information to consumers" (DSHEA, 1994). The DSHEA has received extensive criticism within the medical community for leaving consumers without sufficiently accurate disclosure to make informed decisions regarding herbal products. A secondary criticism has been that the DSHEA allows patients to purchase medicinal substances without prior proof of safety or efficacy. Such criticisms are warranted and have led to calls for increased vigilance—and regulation—to help ensure product safety. At the same time, however, the DSHEA *expressly* articulates a public policy tilt by the Congress, in the domain of dietary supplements, toward consumer autonomy and away from government regulation. Future regulation concerning dietary supplements should account for all the ethical commitments articulated earlier, balancing the interests of competing stakeholders and better accounting for public safety, while enhancing the disclosure necessary to facilitate informed, autonomous choices.

Health care fraud, another important area of legal concern, also is embedded in both federal and a variety of state statutes (such as consumer fraud laws), both civil and criminal, and common-law rules (such as the proscription against misrepresentation). Legally, fraud requires deception as well as the intent to deceive (Cohen, 1995). The concern for fraud pervades regulation of CAM therapies and, indeed, was part of the early rationale for physician licensure (Cohen, 2003). Yet, because the label of "fraud" often has been concluded rather than proven by law and evidence, Congress (in legislative history) has clarified in at least one context— submission of claims for reimbursement by federal and other funds—that the practice of CAM therapies "itself would not constitute fraud" (Report, 1996). Of course, if a practitioner engages in conduct that exploits patients or unjustifiably diverts them from necessary conventional care, such conduct may lead to malpractice liability, professional discipline, or other legal action, even if not necessarily actionable or fraud. *Third-party reimbursement* also implicates legal rules, as notions of "medical necessity" and what constitutes "experimental treatments" may change as integrative health care unfolds (Cohen, 1998). Finally, the *use of spirituality* in clinical settings, whether through biomedical or CAM therapies, also implicates liability and other legal as well as ethical considerations (Cohen, 2003) and requires sensitivity, professionalism, and care to ensure that patients are offered opportunities to draw on spiritual support without being unduly coerced thereby (Koenig, 2002; Cohen, 2003). Once again, considerations of spirituality in clinical settings should be guided by considerations of nonmaleficence, beneficence, autonomy, pluralism, and accountability.

Notably, in reviewing the complex interaction of preeminent ethical commitments and relevant legal rules, the existing legal and regulatory framework emerged from late-nineteenth century rivalries between the "regular" physicians and their economic and ideological competitors (mainly, chiropractors and homeopaths) in the provision of health care services (Kaptchuk and Eisenberg, 2001; Rothstein, 1972; Shryock, 1967; Stevens, 1971; Starr, 1982). These sectarian rivalries shaped a regulatory environment in which CAM providers often struggled for legal acceptance, and in which CAM providers, and physicians utilizing CAM therapies, found varying levels of regulatory oversight and tolerance (Cohen, 1998). A more balanced perspective must incorporate notions of medical pluralism (Kaptchuk and Eisenberg, 2001) in a way that assures more unbiased consideration of other medical traditions and enables more complete representation by consumers and the various professional groups. In sum, to the extent that the medical, social, political, and public health environments are changing, legal and regulatory structures also are changing and may further evolve (Cohen, 2000; Callahan, 2002; Cohen, 2003).

The sectarian rivalries that have shaped the regulatory and legal environment have also been at play in the formation of conventional medicine's ethical precepts. Medicine is and has always been permeated with the culture and values of its time and place, and hence is constantly shaping and being shaped by the larger social, cultural, and political forces of its era. The history of medical ethics over the past 2,500 years is vivid testimony to the ways this has occurred. The prevalence and persistence of CAM therapies is another juncture in this evolution. Without rejecting what has been of great value and service in the past, it is important that ethical norms are brought under critical scrutiny and evolve, along with medicine's expanding knowledge base and the larger social aims and meanings of medical practice.

REFERENCES

AANP (American Association of Naturopathic Physicians). 1990. *Naturopathic Code of Ethics*. [Online]. Available at: http://www.naturopathic.org/positions/ethics.html [accessed June 17, 2004].

ACA (American Chiropractic Association). 1996. *Code of Ethics*. [Online]. Available at: http://www.acatoday.com/about/ethics.shtml [accessed June 17, 2004].

Adams KE, Cohen MH, Eisenberg D, Jonsen AR. 2002. Ethical considerations of complementary and alternative medical therapies in conventional medical settings. *Ann Intern Med* 137(8):660–664.

American College of Physicians, Ad Hoc Committee on Medical Ethics. 1998. Kitchens LW, Snyder L, Morin K, eds. *Ethics Manual*. 4th ed. Philadelphia, PA: American College of Physicians.

Appelbaum PS, Roth LH, Lidz CW, Benson P, Winslade W. 1987. False hopes and best data: Consent to research and the therapeutic misconception. *Hastings Cent Rep* 17(2):20–24.

Astin JA. 1998. Why patients use alternative medicine: Results of a national study. *JAMA* 279(19):1548–1553.

Astin JA, Astin AW. 2002. An integral approach to medicine. *Alternative Therapies in Health & Medicine* 8(2):70–75.

Beauchamp TL, Childress JF. 1994. *Principles of Biomedical Ethics*. 4th ed. New York: Oxford University Press.

Bratman S. 1997. Alternative medicine: How well does it live up to its own ideals? *Altern Ther Health Med* 3(6):128, 127.

Brody H. 2002. The placebo effect: Implications for the Study and Practice of Complementary and Alternative Medicine. In: Callahan D, ed. *The Role of Complementary and Alternative Medicine: Accommodating Pluralism*. Washington, DC: Georgetown University Press. Pp. 74–83.

Callahan D. 1996. Specifying the goals of medicine. *Hastings Center Report* supplement:(9–14).

Callahan D. 2002. *The Role of Complementary and Alternative Medicine Accommodating Pluralism*. Washington, DC: Georgetown University Press.

Churchill LR. 1995. Beneficience. In: Reich WT, ed. *Encyclopedia of Bioethics*. Vol. 1. Revised ed. New York: Simon & Schuster, McMillan. Pp. 243–247.

Churchill LR, Collins ML, King NM, Pemberton SG, Wailoo KA. 1998. Genetic research as therapy: implications of "gene therapy" for informed consent. *J Law Med Ethics* 26(1):38-47, 3.

Cohen MH. 1995. A fixed star in health care reform: The emerging paradigm of holistic healing. *Arizona State L J* 27:79–173.

Cohen MH. 1998. *Complementary & Alternative Medicine Legal Boundaries and Regulatory Perspectives*. Baltimore, MD: Johns Hopkins University Press.

Cohen MH. 1999a. Malpractice considerations affecting the clinical integration of complementary and alternative medicine. *Curr Prac of Med* 2(4):87–89.

Cohen MH. 1999b. Healing at the borderland of medicine and religion: Regulating potential abuse of authority by spiritual healers. *J L & Relg* 18(2):373–426.

Cohen MH. 2000. *Beyond Complementary Medicine Legal and Ethical Perspectives on Health Care and Human Evolution*. Ann Arbor: University of Michigan Press.

Cohen MH. 2003. *Future Medicine Ethical Dilemmas, Regulatory Challenges, and Therapeutic Pathways to Health Care and Healing in Human Transformation*. Ann Arbor: University of Michigan Press.

Cohen MH, Eisenberg DM. 2002. Potential physician malpractice liability associated with complementary and integrative medical therapies. *Ann Intern Med* 136(8):596–603.

Cohen MH, Ruggie MC. 2004. Integrating complementary and alternative medical therapies in conventional medical settings: Legal quandaries and potential policy models. *Cinn L Rev* 72(2):671–729.

Daugherty C, Ratain MJ, Grochowski E, Stocking C, Kodish E, Mick R, Siegler M. 1995. Perceptions of cancer patients and their physicians involved in phase I trials. *J Clin Oncol* 13(5):1062–1072.

Daugherty CK, Banik DM, Janish L, Ratain MJ. 2000. Quantitative analysis of ethical issues in phase I trials: A survey interview of 144 advanced cancer patients. *IRB* 22(3):6–14.

Dresser R. 2002. The ubiquity and utility of the therapeutic misconception. *Soc Philos Policy* 19(2):271–294.

(DSHEA) Dietary Supplement Health and Education Act of 1994. Public Law No. 103-417, 108 Stat. 4325, 21 U.S.C. ss. 301 et seq. 1994.

Eisenberg D. 1997. Advising patients who seek alternative medical therapies. *Annals of Internal Medicine* 127(1):61–69.

Eisenberg DM, Kessler RC, Foster C, Norlock FE, Calkins DR, Delbanco TL. 1993. Unconventional medicine in the United States: Prevalence, costs, and patterns of use. *N Engl J Med* 328(4):246–252.

Eisenberg DM, David RB, Ettner SL, Appel S, Wilkey S, VanRompay M, Kessler RC. 1998. Trends in alternative medicine use in the United States, 1990-1997: Results of a follow-up national survey. *JAMA* 280(18):1569–1575.

Eisenberg DM, Cohen MH, Hrbek A, Grayzel J, Van Rompay MI, Cooper RA. 2002. Credentialing complementary and alternative medical providers. *Ann Intern Med* 137(12):965–973.

Emanuel EJ, Wendler D, Grady C. 2000. What makes clinical research ethical? *JAMA* 283(20): 2701–2711.

Ernst E, Cohen MH. 2001. Informed consent in complementary and alternative medicine. *Arch Intern Med* 161(19):2288–2292.

Fromm-Reichmann F. 1960. *Principles of Intensive Psychotherapy*. 1st ed. Chicago, and London: University of Chicago Press, Phoenix Books.

FSMB (Federation of State Medical Boards). 2002. Model Guidelines for the Use of Complementary and Alternative Therapies in Medical Practice. [Online]. Available: http://www.fsmb.org/Policy%20Documents%20and%20White%20Papers/cam_model_guidelines.htm [accessed January 12, 2005].

Glik DC. 2000. Incorporating Symbolic, Experimental and Societal Realities into Effectiveness Research on CAM. In: Kelner M, Wellman B, eds. *Complementary and Alternative Medicine: Challenge and Change*. Amsterdam, Abingdon: Harwood Academic. Marston. Pp. 195–208.

Henderson G, King NMP. 2003. What subjects and researchers expect and consent forms say about Gene Transfer Research. *Presentation to National Institutes of Health Recombinant DNA Advisory Committee.*

Hilts PJ. 2003. *Protecting America's Health: The FDA, Business, and One Hundred Years of Regulation*. New York: Alfred A. Knopf.

Holmes HB, Purdy LM. 1992. *Feminist Perspectives in Medical Ethics*. Bloomington: Indiana University Press.

Ingerman S. 1991. *Soul Retrieval Mending the Fragmented Self*. 1st ed. San Francisco, CA: Harper, San Francisco.

Jonas WB. 1998. Alternative medicine—learning from the past, examining the present, advancing to the future. *JAMA* 280(18):1616–1618.

Jonas WB. 2002. Policy, the public, and priorities in alternative medicine research. *Annals of the American Academy of Political and Social Science* 583:29–43.

Jonas WB, Chez RA. 2003. Definitions and standards in healing research: First American Samueli Symposium. *Alternative Therapies in Health and Medicine* 9(3 Suppl):A5–A104.

Kaptchuk TJ, Eisenberg DM. 2001. Varieties of healing. 1: Medical pluralism in the United States. *Ann Intern Med* 135(3):189-95.

King NM. 1995. Experimental treatment. Oxymoron or aspiration? *Hastings Cent Rep* 25(4):6–15.

Kleijnen J, Knipschild P. 1992. Ginkgo biloba for cerebral insufficiency. *Br J Clin Pharmacol* 34(4):352–358.

Le Bars PL, Katz MM, Berman N, Itil TM, Freedman AM, Schatzberg AF. 1997. A placebo-controlled, double-blind, randomized trial of an extract of Ginkgo biloba for dementia. North American EGb Study Group. *JAMA* 278(16):1327–1332.

Maslow AH. 1968. *Toward a Psychology of Being*. 2d ed. Princeton, NJ: Van Nostrand: Van Nostrand Insight Books.

Mastroianni A, Kahn J. 2001. Swinging on the pendulum. Shifting views of justice in human subjects research. *Hastings Cent Rep* 31(3):21–28.

Mike V. 1999. Outcomes research and the quality of health care: The beacon of an ethics of evidence. *Eval Health Professions* 22:3–32.

Miller FG, Emanuel EJ, Rosenstein DL, Straus SE. 2004. Ethical issues concerning research in complementary and alternative medicine. *JAMA* 291(5):599–604.

Miller M. 2000. Phase I cancer trials. A collusion of misunderstanding. *Hastings Cent Rep* 30(4):34–43.

Moore v. Baker. 1991. U.S. Dist. LEXIS 14712, at *11 (S.D. Ga., Sept 5, 1991), aff'd, 989 F.2d 1129.

NAFTA Acupuncture and Oriental Medicine Commission. [Online]. Model Code of Ethics. Available at: http://www.nacaom.org/ethics.php [accessed June 17, 2004].

NIH (National Institutes of Health). 1995. Alternative Medicine: Expanding Medical Horizons. A Report to the National Institutes of Health on Alternative Medical Systems and Practices in the United States. Washington, DC: U.S. Government Printing Office.

NIH (National Institutes of Health). 1997. Acupuncture. National Institutes of Health Consensus Development Statement. [Online]. Available: http://odp.od.nih.gov/consensus/cons/107/107_statement.htm [accessed January 12, 2005].

NIH Consensus Conference. Acupuncture. 1998. *JAMA* 280(17):1518–1524.

Orkin SH, Motulsky AG. 1995. *Report and Recommendations of the Panel to Assess the NIH Investment in Resesarch on Gene Therapy*. NIH.

Ornish D. 1998. *Love & Survival: The Scientific Basis for the Healing Power of Intimacy*. 1st ed. New York: HarperCollins. [Online]. Available: http://www.nih.gov/new/panelrep.html [accessed January 12, 2005].

Pellegrino ED, Thomasma DC. 1993. *The Virtues in Medical Practice*. New York: Oxford University Press.

Report on H.R. 3103. 1996. *Health Insurance Portability and Accountability Act of 1996*. 142:115 Cong. Rec. H9537-38.

Ritvo P, Irvine J, Katz J, Matthew A, Sacamano J, Shaw BF. 1999. The patient's motivation in seeking complementary therapies. *Patient Educ Couns* 38(2):161–165.

Rosen SM. 1982. David Bohm's "Wholeness and the Implicate Order": An interpretive essay. *Man-Environment Systems* 12(January):9–18.

Ross G, Erickson R, Knorr D, Motulsky AG, Parkman R, Samulski J, Straus SE, Smith BR. 1996. Gene therapy in the United States: A five-year status report. *Hum Gene Ther* 7(14):1781–1790.

Rothstein WG. 1972. *American Physicians in the Nineteenth Century: From Sects to Science*. Baltimore, MD: Johns Hopkins University Press.

Shryock RH. 1967. *Medical Licensing in America, 1650-1965*. Baltimore, MD: Johns Hopkins Press.

Starr P. 1982. *The Social Transformation of American Medicine*. New York: Basic Books.

Stevens R. 1971. *American Medicine and the Public Interest*. New Haven, CT: Yale University Press.

Studdert DM, Eisenberg DM, Miller FH, Curto DA, Kaptchuk TJ, Brennan TA. 1998. Medical malpractice implications of alternative medicine. *JAMA* 280(18):1610–1615.

Sugarman J, Burk L. 1998. Physicians' ethical obligations regarding alternative medicine. *JAMA* 280(18):1623–625.

Thorne S, Best A, Balon J, Kelner M, Rickhi B. 2002. Ethical dimensions in the borderland between conventional and complementary/alternative medicine. *J Altern Complement Med* 8(6):907–915.

Thurman RAF. 1998. *Inner Revolution: Life, Liberty, and the Pursuit of Real Happiness*. New York: Riverhead Books.

Truant T, McKenzie M. 1999. Discussing complementary therapies: There's more than efficacy to consider. *CMAJ* 160(3):351–352.

U.S. Advisory Committee on Human Radiation Experiments. 1996. *Final Report of the Advisory Committee on Human Radiation Experiments*. New York: Oxford University Press.

United States v. Rutherford. 438 F. Supp. 1287 (W.D. Okla. 1977), Remanded, 582 F.2d 1234 (10th Cir. 1978), Rev'd, 442 U.S. 544 (1979), on Remand, 616 F.2d 455 (10th Cir. 1980), Cert. Denied, 449 U.S. 937 (1980), Later Proceeding, 806 F.2d 1455 (10th Cir. Okla. 1986).

U.S. House of Representatives. 1996. Hearing of the Oversight and Investigations Subcommittee of the House Commerce Committee on Access to Medical Treatment.

Young JH. 1992. *American Health Quackery: Collected Essays*. Princeton, NJ: Princeton University Press.

7

Integration of CAM and Conventional Medicine

A distinct trend toward the integration of complementary and alternative medicine (CAM) therapies with the practice of conventional medicine is occuring. Hospitals are offering CAM therapies, health maintenance organizations (HMOs) are covering such therapies, a growing number of physicians use CAM therapies in their practices, insurance coverage for CAM therapies is increasing, and integrative medicine centers and clinics are being established, many with close ties to medical schools and teaching hospitals. How does a new therapy move from the idea stage to the practice stage? What is the extent of integration of CAM and conventional medicine? Why is such integration occurring? What approaches are being used to offer integrated services? This chapter explores these and other questions related to the integration of CAM and conventional medicine.

FROM IDEA TO PRACTICE

Ideally, conventional medical tests and treatments go through a series of scientific challenges that, if met, allow the test or the treatment to become part of conventional medical practice. However, there are and there always will be exceptions. As noted in Chapter 4, some new practices offer dramatic and evident benefits that may justifiably hasten their acceptance. Sometimes, enthusiasm for the intervention, founded on the plausibility of the benefits and the absence of satisfactory alternatives, speeds acceptance, despite a dearth of evidence (e.g., screening for and treatment of prostate cancer).

Because the emphasis on evidence-based decision making is relatively new, many current conventional medical practices did not follow what is now considered to be the normative pathway of translation because they became accepted practice before this pathway was fully established. Many practices that are widely accepted, however, continue to undergo scrutiny, and their indications often change as research identifies those patients who benefit the most from them. An example is coronary bypass surgery which became accepted treatment before undergoing controlled clinical trials. The evident effectiveness of coronary bypass surgery in reducing symptoms of stable angina fostered great enthusiasm for the procedure, with many clinicians assuming that its effectiveness would be similar in reducing the risks of heart attack and death because of coronary disease. When bypass surgery was already well established, a number of RCTs showed that it improved the life expectancies of patients with severe coronary artery disease but had little effect on patients with mild disease. In addition, it had no effect on heart attack rates. Similarly, patients with acute coronary syndromes that threatened to evolve into myocardial infarction received percutaneous coronary interventions long before RCTs showed that this strategy was superior (by a small margin) to thrombolysis with drugs.

In this idea pathway, the acceptance of new interventions in clinical practice depends on a cycle (Figure 7-1) that begins with a creative idea derived from either an advance in science or a clinical observation. That creative insight is the basis for hypotheses about treatment effectiveness. Hypotheses are tested through a series of evaluation steps before they are accepted, first by early adopters and then more widely. As acceptance grows, a number of forces shape the level of integration of the intervention into clinical practice. These forces may include difficulty in acquiring technical skills, the supply of practitioners or the capacity to deliver the intervention, and coverage decisions made by health plans and other payers. Patient demand for services also affects acceptance and integration. Patient demand is influenced by evidence of effectiveness, but it is also influenced

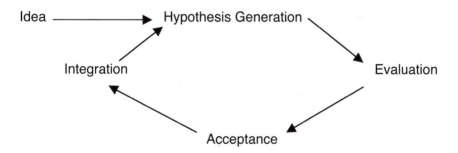

FIGURE 7-1 Translation: from idea to practice.

by individual experience with the treatment and the presence or absence of satisfactory alternatives. After its acceptance, ongoing questioning of the value of an intervention relative to those of other new and established interventions is necessary to refine clinical practice and generate new creative ideas that lead to further clinical advances.

The number of steps or challenges has increased over the past several decades. The process will evolve further, and as the nation looks forward to a health care system in which conventional practice and CAM coexist in close harmony, these processes will apply to new tests and treatments from both the traditions of practice. Several factors are noteworthy, however. First, the series of steps represents a logical progression; however, the process is not uniformly followed in conventional medicine. Second, most existing CAM therapies already exist in practice; that is, patients are using these therapies. This means that the cycle must begin at the integration step so that studies can be carried out to evaluate the therapies already in use. Third, new measures and methods must be developed to adequately reflect patients' experiences with CAM as well as the outcomes most relevant to current users. For therapies that are not well supported by empirical evidence, studies addressing general questions of treatment effectiveness may be most appropriate. For therapies that are well supported, studies that address the underlying mechanisms of action, that identify subgroups of patients in whom the treatment works more or less well, or that test modifications to a general approach to treatment may be appropriate. These steps are not linear; a therapy may be involved in activities at several steps simultaneously, and adoption into practice does not terminate the process. Indeed, the evaluation process continues as new information about a therapy is generated. Given these caveats, a more in-depth exploration of the conceptual model for translation from idea to practice is provided below.

Hypothesis Generation

As noted in Figure 7-1, the first step in the translation process is the generation of an idea. All accepted clinical practices were once just a good idea. The creative insight may have come from a practitioner, a researcher, or even a patient. It may have been derived from an advance in science or from recognition of an unmet clinical need. In any case, once a good idea has become a new treatment, it must be tested.

Evaluation

Once ideas have been generated, they must pass through several stages of evaluation. First, it is necessary to decide which interventions should have priority for evaluation and which types of research designs are best for those evaluations. In effect, research committees at drug companies and National Institutes of Health study sections perform this function by deciding which proposals shall receive funding. The committee suggests that the following criteria (also discussed in Chapter 4) be used when CAM interventions are considered for testing. Clearly, no intervention will meet *all* criteria, and a therapy should not be excluded from consideration because it does not meet any one particular criterion, for example, biological plausibility.

- A biologically plausible mechanism exists for the intervention, with recognition that the science base on which plausibility is judged is a work in progress.
- Research could plausibly lead to the discovery of biological mechanisms of disease or treatment effect.
- The condition is highly prevalent (e.g., diabetes mellitus).
- The condition causes a heavy burden of suffering.
- The potential benefit is great.
- Some evidence already exists that the intervention is effective.
- Some evidence that there are safety concerns exists.
- The research design is feasible and likely to yield an unambiguous result.
- The target condition or the intervention is important enough to have been detected by existing population surveillance mechanisms.

Next in the evaluation part of the cycle is the conduct of preliminary studies to establish feasibility. One example of this process is the Phase I and Phase II trials required by the Food and Drug Administration for new drugs. These studies evaluate whether the intervention does what it claims to and characterizes adverse effects.

If the intervention meets the challenges imposed by the Phase I and II trials, it becomes a candidate for adoption as a medical practice and moves to the next challenge: clinical trials to test its effects with larger numbers of patients.

Acceptance

Several things happen during the acceptance phase of the translation cycle. Once research results are available, dissemination begins. Researchers publish their findings in peer-reviewed journals and make presentations at scientific meetings. This step requires a careful peer-review process and competent researchers to evaluate the evidence and recommend the findings for publication or presentation. The articles may be published in CAM-related journals (e.g., *Journal of Complementary and Alternative Medicine*) and journals that focus on conventional medicine (e.g., *Annals of Internal Medicine* and *New England Journal of Medicine*). Various professional organizations hold scientific sessions at which the investigators present the research results.

After much clinical testing, the accumulating body of evidence provides a basis for strong conclusions about efficacy and effectiveness. At this point, experts on evidence evaluation perform systematic reviews and meta-analyses to estimate the size of the effect of the intervention. These research syntheses form the basis of the next steps. Many syntheses of research on CAM appear, for example, in the Cochrane Collaboration reviews, discussed in Chapter 5.

During the acceptance portion of the cycle, professional organizations and clinical practices also create guidelines to best practices. The American College of Physicians and Kaiser-Permanente are among the organizations that develop guidelines that describe a professional consensus, and these are nearly always based on syntheses of the evidence about best practices.

Payers then decide on coverage policy. Coverage policy is important to the adoption of new tests and treatments, although many patients pay out of pocket for CAM services that payers do not cover. Evaluations may be conducted by an internal group or through a contract with an outside agency. Although the coverage decision is science based (which means that it draws on the findings presented in published studies), it may also be negotiated by providers and major purchasers.

Integration

Once an intervention becomes available for general clinical use, it becomes subject to a process that encourages the adoption of knowledge-based therapies. Factors influencing the adoption of the intervention include use by influential practitioners in the community, ease of use, drug company and device manufacturer sales representatives, advertisements in medical journals, advertisements on television and in other media, presentations and booths at professional meetings, and continuing education events. A more ill-defined process leads to the discarding of technologies that had become established before testing but that fell short of their initial promise when they were subjected to careful clinical testing.

Clinical organizations, often at the behest of payers, develop processes to encourage practitioners to follow best practices. Payers and other organizations create incentives for clinical practitioners to follow best practices and hold them accountable. Once a therapy has been accepted into practice, the cycle does not terminate. As new information is accumulated through practice and additional research, the therapy may be reevaluated.

This conceptual model of how new ideas for interventions move into practice also applies to the integration of CAM and conventional medical therapies, in which many CAM therapies that are new to conventional medicine are being accepted by conventional medical practicioners or integrated into conventional practices. Osteopathic medicine is an example of a discipline that developed separately from conventional medicine, moved through the stages of translation from idea to practice, and is fully accepted as an effective treatment modality. Whorton (2002) describes how Andrew Taylor Still, a frontier physician, founded osteopathy. Still's point of departure for his new system was his view of the body as a machine which should function well if it were mechanically sound. His system was designed to improve health by treating the patient as a whole through improving the circulation and correcting abnormal mechanics. He condemned the prevalent use of drugs by medical practitioners.

In 1892 the first osteopathic school was opened (the American School of Osteopathy), offering training in manipulation as well as classroom instruction in anatomy. Despite resistance by conventional medicine, in 1896 Vermont became the first state to license osteopaths. By the 1920s forty states licensed osteopaths to practice, although it was not until 1973 that osteopathy was licensed in all states.

Some in the osteopathic community argue that osteopathy grew out of a separate tradition, that it has maintained its distinctiveness, and that it should not be considered congruent with conventional medicine. Those who maintain that osteopathy remains a distinct system cite two main reasons: a holistic approach with a focus on preventive care and the "use of osteopathic manipulation as part of the overall therapeutic approach" (Howell, 1999). Others believe that the similarities of osteopathic medicine with conventional medicine greatly outweigh any differences. "Overall, osteopathic medical schools have come to resemble allopathic medical schools in most respects; some students even share classes" (Howell, 1999).

Whether or not osteopathy remains a unique approach to medicine, it has come to be recognized as an effective approach to treatment.

The next section explores trends in the integration of CAM and conventional medicine.

GROWING INTEGRATION OF CAM

In 1998, the American Hospital Association began collecting in its annual survey information about hospitals that offer CAM services and found that only 6 percent of hospitals reported that they offered such CAM services. By 2001, the number of hospitals offering CAM therapies had more than doubled to 15 percent "indicating a steadily growing interest by hospitals to enter into this arena" (Ananth, 2002). HMOs are also increasingly interested in offering CAM therapies. In 1997, Landmark Healthcare,

Inc., commissioned a survey of HMO use of CAM therapies. One hundred fourteen HMOs were surveyed between November 1998 and January 1999, which was 25 percent of all HMOs in existence at the time of the survey. The results showed that two-thirds of HMOs (67 percent) offered at least one form of alternative care, the most common being chiropractic (65 percent) and acupuncture (31 percent) (Landmark Healthcare, Inc., 1999).

Cancer treatment centers also frequently use CAM therapies. Three such programs are briefly described here. The Memorial Sloan-Kettering Cancer Center has developed an Integrative Medicine Service that offers inpatients music therapy, massage therapies and reflexology, and mind-body therapies. Outpatient services include "massage, acupuncture, reflexology, meditation, self-hypnosis and other mind-body therapies, music and sound therapies, and counseling in nutrition and herb-drug issues, as well as classes in yoga, tai chi, chair aerobics, the Alexander technique, Pilates mat, etc." (Cassileth, 2002).

The University of Texas M.D. Anderson Cancer Center supports an integrative medicine program that incorporates research, education, and a clinical program. That facility, called "*Place . . . of wellness,*" opened in 1998. "*Place . . . of wellness* offers more than 75 complementary therapy program opportunities, free of charge, to help with the non-medical issues of living with cancer. It is a bridge between standard medical care and spiritual healing that we call complementary and integrative medicine" (M.D. Anderson Cancer Center, 2004). Therapies include mind-body approaches such as guided imagery and progressive relaxation; physical therapies such as yoga, tai chi, massage, and acupuncture; and nutritional support.

The Dana-Farber Cancer Institute has established the Zakim Center for Integrated Therapies. The center defines integrated therapies as "individual treatments that are used in addition to (or as a complement to) traditional cancer treatment such as chemotherapy and radiation" (Dana-Farber Cancer Institute, 2004). Therapies include massage therapy, acupuncture, and nutritional guidance. The center's website states, "When patients integrate these therapies into their medical and surgical care, they are creating a more comprehensive treatment plan and helping their own bodies to regain health and vitality" (Dana-Farber Cancer Institute, 2004).

In addition, a nonprofit organization of health professionals, the Society for Integrative Oncology (SIO), was created in 2003 to provide "a convenient forum for presentation, discussion, and peer review of evidence-based research and treatment modalities in the discipline known as integrative medicine" in cancer care. (SIO, 2004).

Use of CAM by Conventional Practitioners

Several efforts have been made to examine the extent to which CAM services are being incorporated into physicians' practices. Berman and colleagues (1995) surveyed physicians' attitudes toward CAM and found a high interest in such services. Furthermore, they found that some therapies were already being used by the responding physicians. Of the 180 respondents, more than 90 percent considered legitimate medical practices to include diet and exercise, behavioral medicine, biofeedback, and counseling or psychotherapy. In addition 50 percent believed that acupuncture, massage therapy, and hypnotherapy were legitimate medical practices. Blumberg et al. (1995) surveyed primary care internists and board-certified family physicians and found that of the 572 respondents, more than half would "encourage patients who raise the possibility" of using CAM. Furthermore, 57 percent indicated they would refer their patients for treatment.

Gordon and colleagues (1998) surveyed adult primary-care physicians and obstetrics-gynecology physicians and nurse practitioners from a large northern California HMO. During the 12 months before the survey, "90 percent of adult primary care physicians and obstetrics-gynecology clinicians recommended at least one alternative therapy." Table 7-1 provides the percentages by type of therapy.

Another survey by Berman and colleagues (1998) found that almost 20 percent of the physicians had used in their practice 9 of the therapies listed in Table 7-2 and that one-third or more were open to using 17 of them. Table 7-2 displays the percentage of physicians who have incorporated various CAM modalities or who would do so.

A review of the literature by Astin et al. (1998) found that "large numbers of physicians are either referring to or practicing some of the more prominent and well-known forms of CAM and that many physicians believe that these therapies are useful or efficacious." Analysis across surveys revealed that the rates of physician referral were 43 percent for acupuncture, 40 percent for chiropractic, and 21 percent for massage, with about half of the physicians indicating belief in the efficacies of these therapies. For homeopathy and herbal approaches, 26 and 23 percent of physicians, respectively, believed in the efficaces of these therapies.

In recognition of the growing use of CAM therapies by individual conventional medical practitioners, the Federation of State Medical Boards of the United States developed *Model Guidelines for the Use of Complementary and Alternative Therapies in Medical Practice*. The guidelines focus on "encouraging the medical community to adopt consistent standards, ensuring the public health and safety by facilitating the proper and effective use of both conventional and CAM treatments, while educating physicians

TABLE 7-1 Alternative Therapies Being Used or Recommended by Adult Primary-Care and Obstetrics-Gynecology Clinicians for Patient Care

Alternative Therapy	Percentage of Adult Primary-Care Clinicians (n = 624)	Percentage of Obstetrics-Gynecology Clinicians (n = 157)
Manipulation therapies	72.9	68.1
Chiropractic	33.6	37.6
Osteopathy	5.1	5.7
Acupuncture	57.2	42.7
Acupressure	30.9	30.6
Massage therapy	42.5	44.6
Body work	7.5	12.1
Ingested therapies[a]	29.5	54.1
Herbal or botanical medicine	8.8	29.3
Homeopathic medicine	2.7	9.5
Special diet	18.3	28.0
Megadoses of vitamins, etc.	8.3	21.7
Mind-body therapies	74.8	70.7
Meditation, mindfulness	48.9	45.8
Relaxation techniques	67.6	63.7
Guided imagery, visualization	16.7	22.9
Biofeedback	31.9	22.9
Hypnosis, self-hypnosis	11.5	14.0
Movement therapies	27.7	26.1
Yoga	19.5	22.9
Tai chi, chi gong	17.9	10.2
Supportive therapies	84.9	80.2
Religious healing or prayer	13.6	12.7
12-step program, support group	58.0	48.4
Psychological counseling	78.7	77.1

[a]Many of the clinicians who indicated that they used or recommended a special diet described the type only as "low fat" or "low sodium." Thus, the prevalence reported for this modality is likely inflated by providers who recommended more conventional diets for patients with heart disease, diabetes mellitus, or hypertension. Excluding special diet, the proportions of clinicians who reported that they recommended ingested therapies are 16.3 percent for adult primary-care physicians and 42.0 percent for obstetrics-gynecology clinicians.

SOURCE: Gordon et al. (1998).

on the adequate safeguards needed to assure these services are provided within the bounds of acceptable professional practice" (FSMB, 2002).

Nurses also use CAM therapies in their practices. Sparber (2001) presented the results of an investigation of State Boards of Nursing (BONs) positions on nurses' practice of CAM therapies and found that 47 percent

TABLE 7-2 Percentage of Physicians Who Have Used or Who Would Use CAM Practices, by Specialty (n = 783)

Practice	Total Sample Have Used	Total Sample Would Use	Total	Pediatrics	Internal Medicine	Family and General Practice
Diet, exercise	92.3	6.5	98.8	98.9	99.1	98.4
Counseling, psychotherapy	71.2	24.5	95.7	96.1	94.8	96.1
Behavioral medicine	47.3	43.8	91.1	92.6	91.5	92.5
Biofeedback, relaxation	44.1	47.6	92.7	92.1	91.5	92.5
Massage, therapeutic touch	33.7	30.9	64.6	51.7	62.5	72.5
Prayer, spiritual direction	29.2	32.4	61.6	57.6	59.9	65.1
Vegetarianism	24.0	39.0	63.0	55.1	63.8	66.9
Meditation	24.0	42.8	66.8	57.6	65.1	73.2
Hypnotherapy	19.9	48.0	67.9	62.9	65.7	71.2
Chiropractic	19.2	29.0	48.2	32.9	50.6	54.5
Megavitamin	16.2	21.3	37.5	18.9	38.7	45.9
Acupuncture	11.7	48.7	60.4	47.7	68.9	60.7
Acupressure	10.1	36.5	46.6	30.1	44.6	56.6
Herbal medicine	8.2	34.3	42.5	34.2	43.6	46.1
Homeopathic medicine	5.9	27.9	33.8	26.3	29.4	41.2
Art therapy	5.0	39.5	44.5	44.6	42.8	44.5
Electromagnetic applications	3.8	20.6	24.4	18.2	21.9	27.2
Native American medicine	2.8	29.8	32.6	26.4	33.9	34.9
Traditional Oriental medicine	2.4	33.5	35.9	29.4	38.1	37.6

SOURCE: Adapted from Berman et al. (1998).

of the BONs permitted nurses to practice a range of CAM therapies and an additional 13 percent were in the process of discussing whether to allow nurses to perform such therapies. The Minnesota Board of Nursing has developed a statement of accountability with several specific points on the use of CAM in nursing. The document states, "[N]urses who employ integrative therapies in their nursing practice to meeting nursing and patient goals developed through the nursing process are held to the same accountability for reasonable skill and safety as they are with the implementation of conventional treatment modalities"(Minnesota Board of Nursing, 2003). The Gillette Nursing Summit, held in May 2002, was convened to "identify common concerns and a set of core recommendations that would enable nurses to provide leadership in this emerging field" of integrated health and healing (Kreitzer and Disch, 2003) and resulted in the development of recommendations related to integrated health care in the areas of research, education, clinical care, and policy. Tracy et al. (2003) evaluated nurses' attitudes toward CAM use in critical care and found that nurses are open to the use of CAM therapies, with many already incorporating CAM therapies into their own practices. Kreitzer et al. (2002) questioned medicine, nursing, and pharmacy faculty and students at the University of Minnesota and found that "more than half of the medical and nursing faculty either would personally provide or refer a CAM practitioner for acupuncture, biofeedback, chiropractic, hypnosis or guided imagery, massage, and meditation. . . . Pharmacy faculty were less likely to provide CAM therapies or refer [a patient] to a CAM practitioner, though more than 50 percent would do so for herbal medicine and nutritional supplements and more than 40 percent for acupuncture, chiropractic, massage, or prayer or spiritual healing."

Reimbursement for CAM Services

Coverage of CAM services is an important issue for the integration of conventional medicine and CAM. In 1999 a study examining insurance coverage of CAM services was conducted in New York, New Jersey, and Connecticut. "Virtually all of the insurance carriers in the survey cover chiropractic services in some form," almost 40 percent (17 of 43) cover acupuncture, and 37 percent (16 of 43) cover massage therapy (Cleary-Guida et al., 2001). Weeks (1999) found that although the extent of CAM integration into benefit designs in early 1999 was "extremely limited," most national plans either had a CAM product or a CAM strategy team. The different coverage options identified by Weeks appear in Table 7-3.

Weeks (2001) concluded in another article that "The dominant trend during 1998 to 2000 . . . was a conservative move to offer CAM through discounted, value-added affinity programs. When plans actually cover CAM

TABLE 7-3 CAM Coverage Offered by Some Insurance Policies

Insurance plans offer different levels or types of coverage for CAM services:

Offer CAM, but only subsequent to a state mandate, and therefore without any internal, proactive process

Include direct access to numerous CAM services, but only for workers' compensation claims

Have CAM services, but in only one or two of perhaps two dozen distinct insurance or HMO "products" that it offers to purchasers

Promote a CAM program, but only to its group purchasers and not to individuals

Administer an insurance policy for a self-insured company that has some CAM coverage, but the plan does not offer the coverage

Allow conventional medical providers to offer certain CAM therapies but not cover those services when they are provided by members of distinct CAM professions

Have an offering for which the purchaser must pay more (rider) and that is outsourced to a CAM network but has little to no internal expertise in CAM

Create a program that allows members to access CAM services on a discounted basis but not as a covered benefit

Cover a certain provider category, such as chiropractor, for only very limited conditions, such as low back pain

SOURCE: Weeks (1999).

services, most do so as an added benefit contracted by employers or groups through insurance riders with services provided at an added cost and through credentialed networks of practitioners." In this context, it is noteworthy that Wolsko et al. (2002) found that the extent of insurance coverage for CAM providers and the use of CAM therapies for wellness are strong correlates of the frequent use of CAM providers. Furthermore, about 8.9 percent of the U.S. population was responsible for more than 75 percent of the visits to CAM providers.

It should be noted that not all CAM practitioners are convinced that insurance coverage is positive for the future practice of complementary and alternative medicine. Cleary-Guida et al. (2001) cautioned that "the consequences of including CAM services in health insurance plans are unknown and require careful consideration." One concern is whether the quality of and levels of reimbursement for CAM services will deteriorate once they are covered by health insurance and subjected to the limitations imposed by carriers or the restrictions of managed care organizations. Other practitioners believe that CAM "will never fulfill its promise if it cannot be delivered via direct pay insurance" (Clohesy Consulting, 2003). Between these extremes are those who believe that it is possible to maintain the desire of integrative medicine for a system of relationship-based care yet also for CAM services to qualify for insurance reimbursement.

The data presented above indicate that hospitals, managed care organizations, and conventional practitioners have incorporated some CAM therapies into the provision of health care services. The next section discusses what is known about the reasons for integration of CAM and conventional medicine.

WHY IS INTEGRATION OCCURRING?

The reasons why *individuals* choose to use CAM therapies were explored in Chapter 2. Although few studies have focused on why health care institutions and practioners are incorporating CAM therapies, this section examines the available evidence about why institutions and practitioners (both conventional medicine and CAM) are moving toward integrated care.

The American Hospital Association survey of hospitals found that 49 percent of respondents indicated that patient demand was the primary motivation for offering CAM services, whereas another 24 percent stated that offering these services reflected their organizational mission. Survey respondents stated other motivators for offering CAM: clinical effectiveness (45 percent), attracting new patients (41 percent), and differentiation from competitors (36 percent). Major obstacles to implementing successful CAM programs included physician resistance (63 percent), budgetary constraints (52 percent), lack of internal expertise (39 percent), and credentialing of providers (33 percent). The survey also found that the principal form of payment for hospital-based CAM services is patient self-pay (76 percent) (Ananth, 2002).

In the Landmark Healthcare, Inc. (1999) survey of HMOs, the respondents indicated that their reasons for offering alternative care were market, employer, or consumer demand (71 percent); the effectiveness of the therapies (29 percent); or state mandates or legal requirements (29 percent). The most important factors that HMOs take into account when they evaluate CAM providers are quality of care, the credentials and qualifications of the providers, and price competitiveness (Landmark Healthcare, Inc., 1999).

As part of a literature review and survey designed to determine which insurers had special policies for CAM coverage and which hospitals were offering CAM, Pelletier et al. (1997) determined that "consumer demand for CAM is motivating more insurers and hospitals to assess the benefits of incorporating CAM." Follow-up studies in 1998 and 1999 produced similar results. Weeks (1999) examined the forces shaping CAM coverage, the extent of coverage offered by insurers and health care plans, and models for inclusion or coverage and found that key motivators for CAM inclusion are "mission, marketplace, mandates, and medicine."

Few studies have specifically focused on why physicians are increasingly interested in and positive about CAM. Some evidence, indicates, however, that physicians want to know more about CAM to better "keep up with their patients' growing interest in and use of CAM" (Ruggie, 2004). Corbin Winslow and Shapiro (2002) found that 84 percent of physicians thought that they needed to learn more about CAM. The strongest reason for this was so that they could better communicate with their patients about the use of CAM. In addition, physician recommendation of CAM (48 percent) was most strongly associated with physician CAM self-use, with physicians who used one or more CAM therapies being seven times more likely to recommend CAM to their patients.

Sikand and Laken (1998) found that sex, ethnicity, practice type, and location of medical training have a significant effect on pediatricians' attitudes toward CAM therapies. Female physicians were found to have more favorable attitudes toward CAM than male physicians, and white physicians where found to have more favorable attitudes than physicians of color. Graduates of U.S. medical schools also had more favorable attitudes toward CAM than their foreign-born or -trained physicians. Blumberg et al. (1995) found that physician involvement in CAM was likely to be higher among younger or female physicians, physicians practicing in the western United States, and family practitioners than among the internists surveyed.

Some hypothesize that conventional medical practitioners are incorporating CAM because of frustrations with the constraints of practice, such as a lack of time necessary for a meaningful patient-practitioner interaction or a loss of autonomy in practice (Snyderman and Weil, 2002). Others suggest that some practitioners, frustrated with a lack of interventions to reduce the effects of chronic conditions (reported to be the leading cause of illness, disability, and death [IOM, 2001]), may be turning to CAM therapies that emphasize prevention and wellness.

Few would argue against the notion that health care practitioners desire to provide the best care for their patients. Some restrict the definition of "best care" to those therapies found in conventional medicine; however, the growing body of evidence demonstrating that some CAM therapies are safe and effective is likely to be a factor contributing to the increased use of CAM by both health care practitioners and health care institutions. Such incorporation is often referred to as *integrative medicine*. The next section explores the emerging approach to health care frequently called *integrative medicine*.

INTEGRATIVE MEDICINE

Integrative medicine is described as more than just the sum of conventional medicine plus CAM. Maizes et al. (2002) defines *integrative medicine* as "healing-oriented medicine that reemphasizes the relationship between patient and physician, and integrates the best of complementary and alternative medicine with the best of conventional medicine." Berndtson (1998) defines the term somewhat similarly, placing emphasis on use of evidence. He writes "integrative medicine refers to a clinical approach that combines the strengths of conventional and alternative medicine with a bias toward options that are considered safe, and which, upon review of the available evidence, offer a reasonable expectation of benefit to the patient."

According to Snyderman and Weil (2002), integrative medicine is a movement, driven by consumers, which is attracting the attention of academic health centers. They write that the focus of integrative medicine is on health and healing and agree with Maizes that the patient-physician relationship is key. They further state, "integrative medicine focuses on preventive maintenance of health by paying attention to all relative components of lifestyle, including diet, exercise, stress management, and emotional well-being. It insists on patients being active participants in their health care as well as on physicians viewing patients as whole persons—minds, community members, and spiritual beings, as well as physical bodies. Finally, it asks physicians to serve as guides, role models, and mentors, as well as dispensers of therapeutic aids."

Hess (2002) views integration as a process that involves a spectrum of options. In his view, at one end of the spectrum (strong integration), patients, under the care of a qualified health professional, are allowed to replace conventional therapies with other options. "At the 'weak' end of the integration spectrum, choices are mostly adjuvant to conventional therapeutic packages. . . . The difference corresponds roughly to the tradeoff in medical ethics between autonomy and paternalism."

Integrative medicine may also be a response to the growing recognition of health professionals that many factors contribute to the health of individuals and the public. Why some people are healthy and others are not has to do "not only with disease and illness, but also with who we are, where we live and work, and the social and economic policies of our government" (IOM, 2003b). This statement reflects the evolution in thinking about health and its determinants that has occurred over the past 50 years. Until about the middle of the twentieth century, health was measured using negative indicators, e.g., mortality and disease rates. Populations with higher mortality rates were considered less healthy than those with lower rates. Such rates continue to be broad indicators of the health of a society.

Efforts to redefine health in the 1950s, however, were spurred by the World Health Organization view of health as "a state of complete physical, mental, and social well being, and not merely the absence of disease or infirmity" (WHO, 1948). This broadened view of what constitutes health led to a rethinking about the determinants of health and how to measure those determinants. According to Bausell and Berman, Engel argued that the context in which the patient operates must be taken into account, that is, a biological, sociological, and psychological model of health should be used (Bausell and Berman, 2002). Lalonde (1974) described a framework of determinants that included environment, lifestyle, human biology, medical care, and health care organization. Evans and Stoddart (1994) developed a more complex model that distinguished among disease, health, functioning, and well-being, arguing that both behavioral and biological responses to the social and physical environments should be included in the understanding of what contributes to health or the lack thereof. A 1999 Institute of Medicine (IOM) report described a model of determinants that showed how individual characteristics and environmental characteristics influence health-related quality of life.

Two recent IOM reports (2003a,b) encourage the use of an *ecological* model of health, that is, a model of health that emphasizes the linkages and relationships among multiple factors (or determinants) affecting health (Figure 7-2). "An ecological model assumes that health and well being are affected by *interaction* among multiple determinants including biology, behavior, and the environment" (IOM, 2003b). The report also states that "an ecological *approach* to health is one in which multiple strategies are developed to impact determinants of health relevant to the desired health outcomes." This ecological approach has some similarities to what CAM practitioners refer to as a *holistic* approach to care.

According to Tauber (2002, p.185), holism was first defined in 1926 by Jan Smuts in a publication called *Evolution and Holism*. As applied to medicine, holism "refers not only to the relational character of medical description and therapy but to the scope of the medical gaze." Ruggie (2004) reports that in the 1970s the word *holistic* referred to health care practices based on the interconnectedness of mind and body. Bausell and Berman (2002), reporting on a study by Barrett et al. (2000), describe holism as representing "a belief in the importance of basing treatment upon people as whole individuals, of taking a multidimensional view of illness, and of trying to get to the heart of the problem rather than simply treating symptoms."

The key point in all these definitions is similar to the idea of the ecological approach, that is, multiple factors influence the health of an individual, and health care practitioners should consider each of these factors in attempting to understand and improve health.

As discussed earlier in this chapter, the level of integration of conventional and CAM therapies is growing. That growth generates the need for tools or frameworks to make decisions about which therapies should be provided or recommended, about which CAM providers to whom conventional medical providers might refer patients, and the organizational structure to be used for the delivery of integrated care. The committee believes that the overarching rubric that should be used to guide the development of

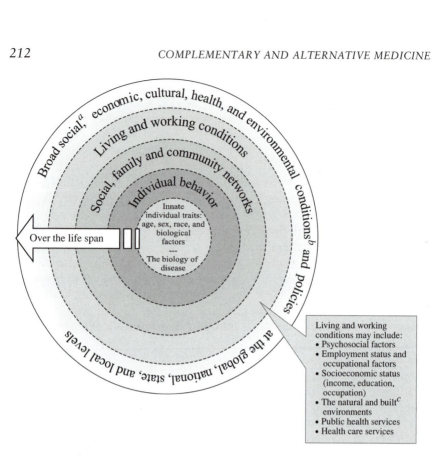

FIGURE 7-2 A guide to thinking about the determinants of population health.

NOTE: The dotted lines between the different levels of the model denote interaction effects between and among the various levels of health determinants (Worthman, 1999). [a]Social conditions include, but are not limited to, economic inequality, urbanization, mobility, cultural values, attitudes, and policies related to discrimination and intolerance on the basis or race, gender, and other differences. [b]Other conditions at the national level might include major sociopolitical shifts, such as recession, war, and governmental collapse. [c]The built environment includes transportation, water and sanitation, housing, and other dimensions of urban planning.

SOURCE: *The Future of the Public's Health* (IOM, 2003a).

these tools should be the goal of providing comprehensive care that is safe and effective, that is collaborative and interdisciplinary, and that respects and joins effective interventions from all sources. Chapters 3, 4, and 5 addressed issues of efficacy and effectiveness and provided a framework for decision making that states that the same principles of evidence and standards of treatment effectiveness should apply to all treatments, whether they are currently labeled as conventional medicine or CAM. The next section presents a conceptual model for deciding when to translate new therapies (CAM or conventional medicine) into practice.

ADVISING PATIENTS

The committee believes that any framework for decision making should encourage patients and practitioners to engage in shared decision making about treatment. One of the 10 rules outlined in the IOM report *Crossing the Quality Chasm* (2001) is that the patient should be viewed as the source of control. The report states, "Patients should be given the necessary information and the opportunity to exercise the degree of control they choose over health care decisions that affect them. The health system should be able to accommodate differences in patient preferences and encourage shared decision making." Such statements can be applied to the desire for shared decision making about CAM therapies as well as those of conventional medicine.

Eisenberg (1997) recommends a nine-step strategy for advising patients:

1. Ask the patient to identify the principal symptom.
2. Suggest that the patient keep a symptom diary.
3. Discuss the patient's preferences and expectations.
4. Review issues of safety and efficacy.
5. Identify a suitable licensed provider.
6. Provide the patient with key questions to ask the provider during the initial consultation.
7. Schedule a follow-up visit (or telephone call) to review the treatment plan.
8. Follow up to review the response to treatment.
9. Provide documentation.

The fourth step of the process proposed by Eisenberg is a review of the safety and efficacy of the treatment under discussion. At this step Cohen and Eisenberg (2002) propose that practitioners may wish to guide their recommendations for treatment for both conventional and CAM therapies by evaluating whether the medical evidence:

- supports both safety and efficacy (option A);
- supports safety, but evidence regarding efficacy is inconclusive (option B);
- supports efficacy, but evidence regarding safety is inconclusive (option C); or
- indicates either serious risk or inefficacy (option D).

Thus, within the framework suggested in Chapter 6 of this report, if the medical evidence supports both safety and efficacy (option A), liability is unlikely and clinicians should recommend the therapy; if the medical evidence indicates either serious risk or inefficacy (option D), liability is probable and clinicians should avoid and actively discourage the patient from using the therapy. If the medical evidence supports safety, but evidence regarding efficacy is inconclusive (option B), or if the medical evidence supports efficacy but evidence regarding safety is inconclusive (option C), then clinicians should caution the patient. If the patient chooses to try the therapy despite the cautionary advice the practitioner should continue to monitor both the efficacy and the safety of the therapy. Figure 7-3 portrays the options graphically.

If patients demand and expect to use therapies for which sufficient evidence to justify the practitioner's recommendation is lacking, then, depending on the medical evidence, the practitioner should caution the patient and monitor efficacy (option B), caution the patient and monitor safety (option C), or encourage the patient to avoid the therapy (option D). In general, if patients choose to make their own decisions, against their conventional practitioner's advice, the practitioner should document this in the patient's medical record. From a liability perspective, the more acute and severe the condition is or the more curable the condition is by conventional medical therapies, the more important it is to monitor and, as neces-

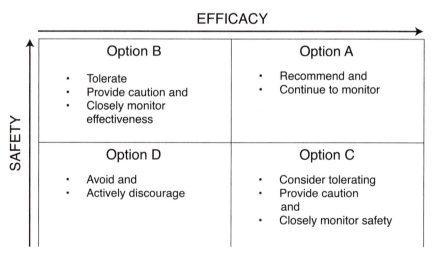

FIGURE 7-3 Clinical risk and the therapeutic posture.
SOURCE: Adapted from Cohen and Eisenberg (2002).

sary, treat the patient by conventional medical practices (Adams et al., 2002; Cohen and Eisenberg, 2002).

The information presented above provides a framework for clinicians. The guidelines developed by the Federation of State Medical Boards also offer information for clinicians to consider (see Appendix E). Conventional medical practitioners should also take into account ethical considerations, as discussed in Chapter 6 when they are advising patients whether to pursue CAM therapies.

Because research regarding both conventional and CAM therapies is ongoing and the medical evidence can change rapidly, the clinician should communicate regularly with the patient regarding any new developments. If, for example, it turns out that high-dose antioxidants negatively interact with chemotherapy, then this information may change the decision to continue the use of high-dose antioxidants during chemotherapy or may change reliance on them as part of a CAM regimen for a period instead of chemotherapy (Cohen and Rosenthal, in press).

If a decision is made to include a therapy provided by another practitioner, the focus of decision making then shifts to identifying practitioners with acceptable expertise. When a patient is referred to a CAM provider, it is important for the conventional medical practitioners to inquire about the provider's training, practice experience, scope of practice, and history of malpractice litigation or professional discipline. Health care institutions are also faced with challenges as they move to consider providing both CAM and conventional medical care. The next section explores issues related to the provision of CAM therapies in health care institutions.

HEALTH CARE INSTITUTIONS

Health care institutions face a number of potential operational barriers to the provision of integrative medicine, including issues of financial sustainability and the development of appropriate clinical models for the provision of medical care by teams comprising various conventional medical and CAM providers. Kreitzer (2001) explored a process for strategic planning and decision making about the inclusion of CAM in existing health care settings. Steps in the planning process include

1. defining who is responsible for gathering information, generating recommendations, and making decisions;
2. identifying and clarifying mandates, both formal (e.g., charters, articles of incorporation and legislation) and informal (tradition or expectations);
3. clarifying the mission and values of the health care system;

4. assessing the external environment for opportunities and challenges (i.e., political climate, economic and social trends, and potential client population); and

5. assessing the internal environment (e.g., people resources and their skills, provider perceptions, and level of interest).

The outcomes from these five steps provide the information necessary for the development of a strategic plan that addresses such issues as whether CAM will be implemented in a systemwide effort or incrementally and whether CAM services will be organized around a core or a center within the system or dispersed throughout the system. Once strategies are developed, all actions and decisions necessary to implement the strategies can be identified (Kreitzer, 2001).

In developing approaches that include both CAM and conventional medical therapies, health care institutions may take advantage of existing health care institution policies and guidelines to address liability concerns, implement risk management practices, and otherwise find ways to appropriately include CAM therapies and providers in existing systems of care. For example, a major area of focus involves credentialing of CAM providers. Such credentialing has parallels to existing hospital mechanisms for credentialing and offering clinical privileges to conventional medical providers; yet credentialing of CAM providers must also incorporate information regarding the standards of education and training, competence, and scopes of practice required by licensing laws in a given state and established by various CAM professional organizations (Eisenberg et al., 2002). Ina (2001) provides guidance for the institutional credentialing process, recommending that source documents should include

- a comprehensive provider application and contract;
- professional license or certification requirements;
- records indicating satisfactory completion of specialty training;
- required professional insurance standards;
- required years of experience;
- peer review of the practitioner's application and all related documents;
- practitioner capabilities for data reporting and profiling; and
- a thorough on-site review of provider offices, records, and operations.

The process of credentialing can be undertaken by the institution itself or through contract with an outside consultant or vendor. According to Ina (2001), 50 percent of organizations surveyed in the report of Landmark